D0500699

# The Firefighter's Workout Book

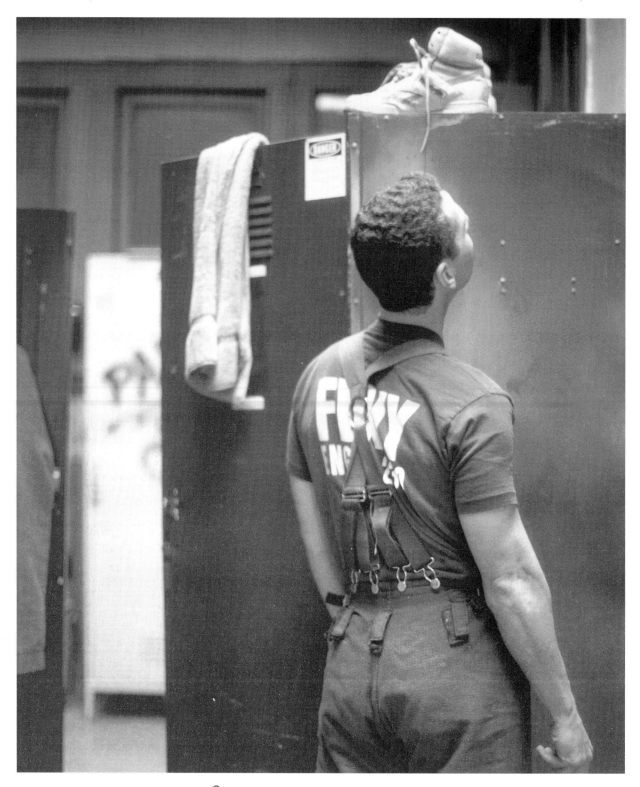

Cliff Street Books
*An Imprint of* HarperCollins*Publishers*

# The Firefighter's Workout Book

## THE 30 MINUTE A DAY

## TRAIN-FOR-LIFE PROGRAM FOR

## MEN AND WOMEN

MICHAEL STEFANO

HarperCollins books may be purchased for educational, business, or sales promotional use. For information please write: Special Markets Department, HarperCollins Publishers Inc., 10 East 53rd Street, New York, NY 10022.

FIRST EDITION

*Designed by Kate Nichols*

Library of Congress Cataloging-in-Publication Data

Stefano, Michael.
    The firefighter's workout book : a 30 minute a day train-for-life program for men and women /
Michael Stefano.
        p.  cm.
     ISBN 0-06-019737-4
     1.  Exercise.    2.  Physical fitness.    I.  Title.
     RA781.S74  2000
     613.7'1—dc21

00-043115

00 01 ❖/ 10 9 8 7 6 5 4 3 2 1

THIS BOOK IS DEDICATED TO

THE MEMORY OF

THE 774 NEW YORK CITY FIREFIGHTERS

WHO HAVE MADE THE SUPREME SACRIFICE

AND DIED IN THE LINE OF DUTY

WHILE PROTECTING

THE CITIZENS OF NEW YORK CITY.

# Contents

# Acknowledgments

I've had a long career, both in fitness and in the fire service. This book has served to tie the two forever together. For me, this project was a labor of love, something that was always within me, but needed to be put down on paper and shared with everyone.

Many people have been involved in the journey and deserve mention here. At the top of the list are my mom and dad, who instilled a sense of perfection in me as a child that has made what's on these pages a true pleasure to read and understand. Next, I'd like to mention Helen, who was at my side all those years with her patience and support, during countless hours of study that sometimes left me no time for the rest of my life.

The workout has been a reality for many years, but putting it down in book form was the original concept of Kelly Hawk, a true visionary and a woman with great ideas. And thanks to Lisa LaPerna, a truly brilliant woman, whose little pushes helped to make this book a reality. My agent, Bob Tabian, deserves special thanks for his recognition of this original idea and his guidance along the way.

Of course, the artistry and sheer visual beauty of the book are credited to two talented artists, Andrew Brucker, the photographer, and Ron DeRosa, the illustrator. Also, a special thanks to all the models involved in the project, firefighters Anthony LaMatina, Steven Lukawski, and Bill Russell, as well as Rebecca Kilgore and Autumn Schmidt. A special mention here goes to my creative consultant, Kim Paolino, whose patience and ability to see beauty in all things are unparalleled. Her support and guidance were endless.

Finally, thank you to the FDNY, and to all the amazing people I've been lucky enough to work with over the years. Special recognition goes to the late firefighter Jim Myerjack, a true pioneer in the fields of firefighting and physical fitness.

# THE FIRE ACADEMY

The New York City fire department is a semimilitary organization, and it runs its training academy like a boot camp. I remember showing up for the first day of training along with the other recruits, the fear of not knowing what to expect written across everyone's face, including mine.

In no time I found myself wrestling with a two-and-a-half-inch-thick high-pressure hose gushing water at over 200 gallons per minute. My arms and shoulders ached as I felt my grip loosen, the water pressure overpowering my most valiant effort to control the hose. I cringed as I heard the training instructor bark out, "More pressure" to the pump operator.

In the weeks to follow I was confronted with many similar situations where I was required to perform under pressure and at my peak capacity. One training evolution after the next tested and taxed all the recruits to the extreme. In addition to operating high-pressure hose lines, we were required to raise and climb heavy ladders, operate superpowerful saws and cutting tools, and rappel down the side of a six-story building—all this while weighted down with bulky protective equipment. My mind and body were being called on to perform like never before, and it was enough to make me realize that the physical and psychological demands of being a firefighter were quite high. Being fit and strong were not an option but a prerequisite to performing the job.

I felt the difference exercise could make. I felt how higher levels of physical endurance made climbing stairs easier, how a stronger upper body could make heavy hoses seem lighter, and how a more tight and toned body made me look and feel years younger than I really was. I made the decision to embrace fitness as a way of life, as a way of coping with life's increased pressures and demands (both mental and physical), and it was one of the best decisions I'd ever made.

# Transformation

**I**n **every person's life** there is a moment that, if seized and acted upon, can transform that person in a profound way. As you've just purchased this book and are embarking upon an exciting new exercise program, this can be one of those transformational moments. You'll begin to understand how your new level of physical fitness will impact every other aspect of your life.

The stronger, more energetic new you will be able to accomplish more with less fatigue. Your interests and hobbies will naturally grow as you find that activities you might have once avoided are now yours for the doing. Whether this means skiing the slopes or just throwing a ball around with your Little Leaguer, life will get sweeter. You'll find you will get sick less often and will sleep better. In fact, exercise physiologists estimate they can slash 10 to 20 years from a physically fit person's *chronological age* when determining his or her *biological age.*

Whether or not you're a firefighter, this book can put you on that path to self-transformation that begins with a healthy, fit body. Just take a minute and ask yourself the following questions:

▶ Are you tired of the image you see when you look in the mirror?

▶ Take an honest look—has your body changed much in the last 5 or 10 years?

▶ Are your clothes fitting differently so that you can't wear the styles you love so much?

▶ Do you tell everyone that your metabolism has slowed down?

▶ Do you want more energy? Do you avoid activities you once embraced?

▶ Are you nagged by constant minor health problems such as colds and flu?

▶ Do constant aches and pains keep you from participating in life?

▶ Are you nagged by chronic minor injuries?

▶ Are life's everyday tasks getting harder and harder?

▶ Do you have trouble falling asleep and even more trouble waking up in the morning?

▶ Or do you have trouble keeping your eyes open during the day?

▶ Do you usually feel stressed out and in a bad mood?

▶ *Do you realize that you can do something about it?*

If you answered yes to any of these questions, you've come to the right place, because this book is all about transformation. The transformation of your entire life is at issue here. Your new and improved physical fitness level will spill over into every other part of your life, including your mental and emotional fitness levels. You'll exude confidence and positive energy. People will begin to perceive you as a confident, capable individual, and everyone will want to know what you've done to look so good.

So you see, this is a really big step, and it's not just about exercise but about taking control of your entire life. I encourage you to take that first step, secure in the knowledge that you cannot fail, because with the *Firefighter's Workout*, a proven, time-tested method to transform the body and mind, results are assured.

Seize the moment, and let's begin the journey together.

## ALL WET

**P**robie is the name the Fire Department of New York (FDNY) gives to its new recruits or rookies. The word *probie* actually stands for *probationary firefighter,* and it's a term every new member knows only too well. Walking through the door of my first firehouse as a probie fresh out of the fire academy, I was ready and willing to do anything that my captain or senior firefighters might ask of me.

The trouble began one night with the first comment about the girth of my arms. "Surely," they mocked, "You look strong enough to do the impossible, like *climb up* the pole that we all slide down." This is great, I so naively thought to myself. Here was my chance to show these guys just how fit and strong I really was (or thought I was). Needless to say, I took the bait and found myself locked in at the bottom of the pole compartment, which was something like a small closet that connected to the second floor by way of a 20-foot polished brass pole.

I took a deep breath and got ready to climb, but the first bucket of water hit me before I could get a hand on the shiny pole, followed by five others in rapid-fire succession. This might have seemed like a frivolous practical joke, but as I stood there like a drowned rat, embarrassed and shivering, I got the message loud and clear: To survive as a firefighter you have to learn to love water, our number-one weapon against almost every fire.

This was the older firefighters' way of acquainting all new recruits with the ever-present possibility of getting soaked (where there's fire, there's water), as well as of making them feel like one of the group. It also prepared probationary firefighters for at least one of the rigors of firefighting—it got them used to being cold and wet, while still being expected to function and to carry out their job.

# The Firefighter's Workout Book

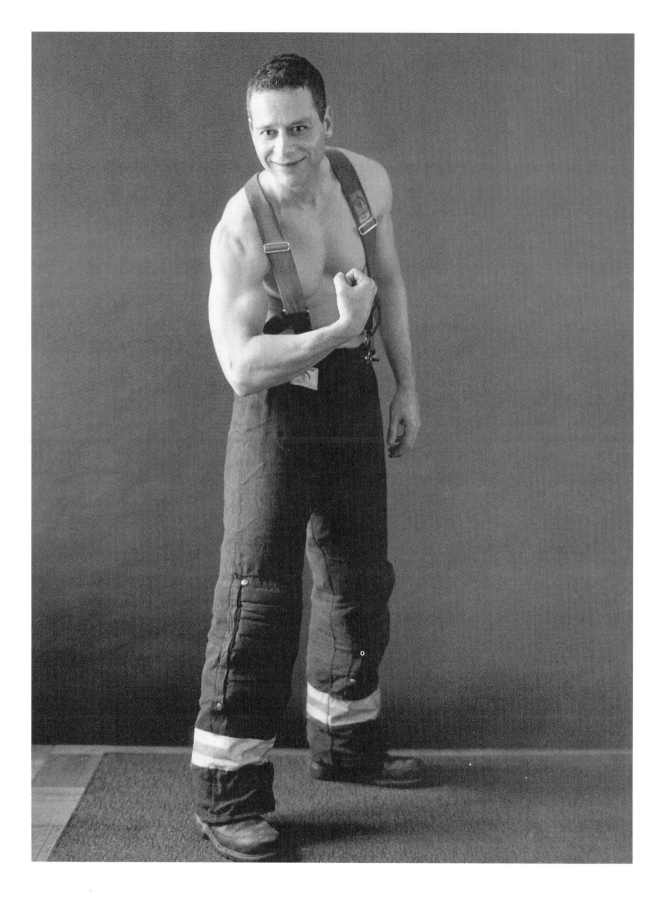

# The Early Days

**W**orking out had always been a way of life for me, so when I began training specifically for the physical aptitude and endurance segment of the New York City firefighters' entrance exam, I didn't have to make that big of an adjustment in my regimen. I set up most of the test events in my parents' backyard and began preparing for the grueling test with the enthusiasm and discipline of an Olympic athlete. My preparation included an obstacle course with an eight-foot wall, a one-mile run, and a 150-pound dummy that had to be carried up a flight of stairs, among other events. I spent many hours preparing for that big day, and it paid off. It was something I really wanted, and I was (and still am) willing to work for it. Thirty thousand people took that test, and fewer than four thousand were actually hired.

What separated the top 10 percent from everyone else were the desire, discipline, and knowledge to get into the kind of shape demanded of a New York City firefighter. If you want to get into shape you face a similar (albeit less grueling) challenge. The desire and discipline must come from you. You've got to reach way down inside yourself and decide what is important in your life right now. Start by asking yourself: *"Are a few hours a week worth having a stronger,* *healthier, leaner body?"* If you're really serious about looking and feeling better, the answer will be a loud and clear, "Yes!"

I can give you the information and knowledge to help you achieve your goals with a minimal amount of time and effort. You heard me—it's unnecessary and even counterproductive to spend hours at the gym or doing endless aerobics. In fact, most firefighters train while at the firehouse, either before or even during their shifts. Usually a long arduous workout isn't even possible between alarms, and the equipment is also often limited. What's needed is a short, rather intense (intense for one's own level of fitness at the time) type of workout that doesn't leave one totally drained and overly fatigued and doesn't require sophisticated or expensive equipment. I needed something that could be accomplished quickly and recovered from just as fast but that would still work. Hence, the Firefighter's Workout was born.

## The Benefits of Exercise

If you can devote four hours a week, you can give yourself the body you've always dreamed of having. Although you might not need the strength and stamina of a firefighter in everyday life, the methods described in this book can still be applied to you. The benefits will be quite the same, and I'll touch on some of those benefits now.

## Increased Strength, Endurance, and Lean Muscle Mass

For the firefighter, the benefits here are obvious. Carrying heavy equipment to the scene of a fire or up many flights of stairs while clad in suffocating, insulated clothing and then being required to perform at full capacity puts tremendous demands of strength and endurance on the human body. For the average individual, life's everyday tasks get easier. Packages begin to feel lighter, and there is suddenly a spring in your step. Your clothes begin to fit differently, and people ask what you've been doing to look so good. Fat melts away, and missing the elevator and taking the stairs doesn't seem like such a big deal any more. Once you get used to this new stronger you, you'll never want to go back.

Worth a mention here is the fact that a strong, lean body is also more efficiently able to cool itself down and warm itself up, making you less susceptible to the ravages of extreme heat or cold. This is absolutely crucial for the working firefighter but also is very important to all Americans, because extremes of temperatures are not uncommon in this country. The trend toward global warming can only worsen this in the years ahead, placing a lot of added stress on the body, especially as we age.

## Increased Flexibility, Range of Motion, Balance, and Coordination

I cannot emphasize enough the importance of a solid flexibility routine as part of your complete workout. Keeping the joints, tendons, ligaments, and muscles limber will prevent injury, period. I've seen it a thousand times in the fire service—the more range of motion you have about a joint, the less chance of

injury when you overextend yourself. Children, the best example of flexibility, appear to be made of clay the way they can bend and twist without injury. While we, as adults, may never again have the flexibility of a 12-year-old child, the fact remains that the more we can bend, the less we'll get hurt.

Flexibility training combined with strength and endurance work also increases athletic performance and circulation, delivering more vital nutrients to the cells of the body. Balance, posture, and body awareness are all enhanced.

## Reduced Cholesterol, Triglycerides, Blood Pressure, Body Fat, and Risk of Disease

The leading cause of line-of-duty death for firefighters across the country is heart attack. While tragic burns and other serious injuries have taken the lives of many brave firefighters, cardiovascular incidents account for almost half of all job-related fatalities. According to an article in the July 1999 issue of *Fire Engineering Magazine*, of the 91 on-duty firefighter deaths across the country in 1998, 39 were the result of heart attacks. We perform our job under the most arduous conditions, enduring high heat and oxygen-deficient environments. Compound this with an intense level of mental stress, and you can see the importance of keeping the cardiovascular system in tip-top shape.

Heart disease is also the leading cause of death for the general public, and what most of us don't realize is that we *all* endure and react to extreme stress in our lives every day, whether it be mental or physical. It's been proven that exercise has a profoundly positive impact on the efficiency of the heart-lung system and its ability to handle these stresses. Exercise also lowers serum cholesterol levels, triglyceride levels, and blood pressure, thereby reducing the risk of heart disease, diabetes, and osteoporosis (a real problem in women as they age), as well as many other ailments. In this modern high-pressure world, you can't afford *not* to work out.

Presented next are three very different examples of the profound effects (both direct and indirect) that exercise can have on people's lives.

## The Comeback Kid

It was dead of winter in the middle of the night when the alarm came in for a store on fire. Lucky Larry was one of the firefighters on duty as the ladder truck raced to the scene. But on that frigid night Larry wasn't so lucky. He was naturally big and strong and, like most firefighters, had been in pretty good shape when he first came on the job. The combination of time taking its toll and a troubled personal life had caused Larry to slip away from his regular exercise program. Not being in the peak physical condition he once had been might have worked against him that night.

Smoke and flame poured from the shattered plate-glass windows as Larry and the rest of the crew arrived. That night, Lucky Larry's assignment was to be part of the "outside team." One of his duties at a fire in this type of structure involved entering the building via a rear door or window and attempting to reach and remove anyone who might still be trapped inside. The big man trotted down an alley, scaled a rickety old fence, and found himself in front of a bare cement wall, the rear wall of the burning store.

In days of old, two ornate oversized windows had provided the rear of the store with light and air, but both openings had since been solidly bricked up, reflecting the security consciousness of the time but now entombing anyone who might be trapped inside. Creating an opening in the rear of the store would also provide much-needed ventilation of the heat and smoke for the crew fighting the fire from inside the store. With urgency in his eyes and adrenaline coursing through his veins, Larry heaved the oversized sledge above his head and swung. Over and over he reached up with the heavy tool and brought it crashing down. Brick by brick, the old window open-

ing gave way—but on one mighty swing, so did Larry's back. His legs buckled, and searing pain brought the big man to his knees.

He spent the next week in the hospital, enduring many tests. It was determined he had severely bulging discs in his lumbar spine. Pain radiated down both legs, and any movement whatsoever was difficult for him. He spent several months in physical therapy and did improve somewhat. His career seemed in jeopardy if he couldn't make better progress by relieving the pain and stiffness enough to function fully as a firefighter.

That's when Larry turned to my program. He needed something beyond physical therapy. Larry's physician outlined the movements he felt the injured firefighter should avoid, and we worked around those limitations. Personally, I felt he needed three things. Number one, more *flexibility*, especially in his lower body. He also needed more *core strength* (strength in the muscles that encase the lower torso, including the abdominal, oblique, and lower back muscles). *Losing weight* would also lighten the load he had to carry.

I sought the advice of my yoga instructor at the time, and we developed a stretching and strengthening routine that didn't aggravate Larry's condition in any way. We suggested a light resistance regimen focusing mostly on the core area. Running was not considered an option due to the stress it places on the lower back. We had to find a cardiovascular exercise intense enough to give Larry a good workout but gentle enough not to aggravate an already bad condition. Walking briskly seemed to work well. A low-fat, highly nutritious diet was suggested to complete the cycle.

Larry spent months on limited duty behind a desk and worked very hard in his off-hours at getting himself strong and pain-free. I was totally impressed with his focus and dedication to his goal of getting back to work. The yoga exercises released tension and restored flexibility and proper alignment where he needed it most. Walking helped melt fat away and reduced the load his injured spinal discs had to withstand. Strength training built a solid foundation around the injured area, further reducing the load the weakened discs had to sustain.

Lucky Larry returned to work that same summer. In the firehouse, you'd find him maintaining the new-found strength and flexibility he'd gained over the previous months. He turned his life around, using his injury as a wake-up call. In addition, he was better able to cope with the problems in his personal life. Luck had nothing to do with his return to work. He demonstrated what discipline, desire, and applied knowledge can do for you, a true success story.

## If You Build It, They Will Work Out

In the dank, damp basement of a 100-year-old firehouse, the firefighters designed and constructed a fully equipped gym. The first problem encountered was water. At times it came right through the building's foundation and seeped everywhere—walls, ceilings, there was absolutely no escaping it. The ingenious solution was to lay an elevated slab of concrete as the gym's floor and form a trough around its perimeter. In the event of any seepage, the water would never reach the elevated slab, but instead would flow harmlessly down the basement drain.

As an extra precaution, a drop ceiling of aluminum was installed. This would effectively channel any water that might drip through the ceiling over the gym to a gutter system and again deliver it harmlessly to the basement drain. In typical New York City firefighter fashion, the water problem was solved.

The next challenge was the funding for the work and for the gym itself. We'd managed to get some funding from the city, and the rest was up to us. How bad did the firefighters want this sorely needed gym? They had to be shown what training could do for them, what a difference it could make in their lives. And I was just the guy to show them. I started a campaign to raise the cash, and everyone was shown the importance of having access to a gym, what it would mean to them, and how it could change their lives.

The idea was to start a firehouse fitness club, which any firefighter could join by paying an initial fee. This initial fee would be minimal, and if members left the firehouse for any reason, they would be compensated with a partial refund. There would be periodic assessments to fund any new equipment or maintenance that might be necessary.

Every one loved the concept, and there was a great response from the firefighters—75 percent joined our fitness club. Fortunately, we were able to get deals on everything from a StairMaster to free weights through one member's connections in the health club industry. Little by little, the gym came together. The members even started to use it on their days off, and everyone was making an attempt at getting fit. Half the battle was won.

Now it was a matter of how to train properly. I consulted with every fitness guru and expert I knew and devised a plan of action. I couldn't be with every firefighter every day as a personal trainer, so I had to get some kind of system down on paper. Sure, I could work with any one individual on any given day, but I had to make provisions for the workouts that couldn't be supervised. It was here that the principles and methods were first recorded.

The idea was to commit the basic principles to paper, allowing for different levels of fitness and fitness goals for each person. Another big consideration was the effect these workouts would have on each firefighter in relation to recovery. Many would be exercising during some downtime (between alarms) while on duty or before their shifts. The workouts couldn't be too time consuming or energy sapping. This applied to resistance as well as cardiovascular training. As a firefighter, you never know what you'll be called on to do in the next five minutes, and you'd better be ready for just about anything. The theory was to keep it short but intense, with quick recovery. Short bursts of intense effort can be more effective than long, arduous training sessions that require extended periods of recovery. The idea was to capitalize on this theory and to create a program that was totally efficient; burned fat; built strength, endurance, and flexibility (vital to protection from injury); and left you energized instead of wiped out. And we wanted to do all this in a period of 30 to 60 minutes. Surely a challenge, but I rose to meet it with the Firefighter's Workout, a complete system for getting in good physical shape in a reasonable amount of time, with a minimal amount of effort.

More important than the new gym itself was the attitude and awareness it fostered in the firefighters. I still firmly believe that you can get a great workout with a little ingenuity and some modest equipment (a good pair of running shoes and a set of dumbbells, for example), but I've got to admit the newly equipped gym got everybody motivated. I printed up an informal version of the workout and issued a copy to each member. In it the methods and principles were all laid out in a simple concise format to meet the goals of each individual. In Chapter 3 of this book, those same basic principles are presented for you to read, understand, and use.

These firefighters, who were confronted with physical and mental challenges almost daily, embraced the opportunity to make their jobs safer and easier as well as to experience the added benefits of losing weight and, looking and feeling better. The program was a total success for them and can be for you, too, today, right now.

## Captain Marathon

He'd completed a dozen New York City Marathons by the time he was 50 years old. He looked 35, and the younger firefighters couldn't keep up with him. With or without my program, this man could run, and he proved it every time the elevators didn't work. In our area of the city, there were many hi-rise apartment houses, better known as housing projects. The status of the elevators in any given building was up for grabs, and most of the structures stood anywhere from 20 to 30 stories. This meant we all did a lot of stair climbing, usually at a pace that would allow us to function after we'd arrived at the right floor.

That day things went a little differently. The big red fire truck pulled up to the building (the address of the reported alarm), and I looked up and saw thick black smoke coming from an apartment on one of the uppermost floors. I donned my air pack, grabbed my tools, and at the same time tried to get a fix on what floor the smoke was coming from. We all raced into the building behind the superfit captain. The first thing he did was hit the elevator call button, and I yelled, "It looks like the twenty-third floor."

We waited no more than one minute, but it felt like an eternity. A thousand different thoughts raced through my head as the captain and I stood staring at each other. Was anyone trapped in the apartment? Would we be able to gain access to the apartment that was on fire? Suddenly there were 10 firefighters in the lobby and no sign of the decrepit old elevator showing any sign of life, so we began the 23-story trek. In gym shorts and sneakers this might not have been too bad, but with full firefighting gear, including an air pack and heavy tools, it was a totally different story.

For the first eight flights, we paced ourselves but managed to keep it brisk. After that, things got a little tougher. The nasty burn in my thighs began to radiate up into my hips, but the captain just kept on going. By the time I'd gotten to the fifteenth floor, I'd lost sight of him. Both my legs had gone numb; I was sweating profusely and breathing very heavily. It was then that I heard this faint voice echoing down the stairwell, and it made me redouble my effort despite the pain. "Were those distant cries for help?" I thought to myself.

I had to completely detach myself from the physical pain I was feeling if I were to have any chance of making it. The faint cries for help grew into piercing screams as I approached floor 23. I knew I couldn't stop. I had to stay with my captain even if I had to crawl up the last two flights, and crawl is just what I did. When I finally arrived on the floor, acrid smoke filled the hallway, and the screams suddenly stopped. I totally didn't expect what happened next.

Like a bat out of hell, the captain rushed past me as I tried to regain enough strength to get back on my feet. He headed toward the stairs, and through the smoke I saw the figure of a young child in his arms. She was slightly injured but conscious as she held onto him for dear life. He carried her down to safety and later explained how he'd found her trapped in a smoky bedroom of the apartment that was on fire and how she'd stopped screaming the minute she looked up at him. He just scooped her up and bolted for the exit while he shared his air supply. Minutes later the rest of the forces arrived with their powerful hoses, and the fire was extinguished rather routinely. There is no doubt in my mind that if it hadn't been for the quick actions of my good captain, the young girl's screams would have been stifled by the choking smoke, not the sight of her rescuer. I found this to be one of the most amazing examples of courage, dedication, and physical and mental stamina I'd ever witnessed.

## Make the Decision to Change

Those early years on the fire department shaped and molded my attitude toward exercise as well as my principles and methods. The firefighters who embraced my program reaped endless benefits, regardless of whether they had to get into shape in order to fight their way back from a serious injury and wanted to safeguard themselves against such events in the future; or they knew the importance of a prime motivator in order to start and stick with a program to achieve their desired goals; or they simply knew that staying in shape was the best way to cope with any challenge that would undoubtedly come their way. These firefighters looked great and performed their jobs even better. The same benefits can be yours.

I met a lot of amazing people at the beginning of my career who achieved dramatic results once they made the decision to change. You see, it's all about making that decision and then going out and finding a system that doesn't waste your time and effort. If you've purchased this book, you're thinking about making that decision right now. I encourage you to go ahead and make it. Take that first step and change your entire life. The Firefighter's Workout presented in the chapters to follow is a tested system of diet and exercise that works. Not only does it work, but it also won't require that you live at the gym in order to accomplish your goals and see results.

I won't promise you a totally new body in six weeks because that's not realistic. Be wary of trainers or books that promise a total new you in no time. They'll say anything to make a sale. If you follow my program, you'll lose fat and build muscle at a rate that's consistent with both a healthy lifestyle *and* reality. I can promise that in about three months' time you'll see a *major difference* in the way your body looks and feels, as well as in your level of fitness. And if you stay with the diet and workout program, the sky's the limit. Of course, the final results will always be up to you. You decide when to shift to a maintenance routine or when you've reached your goals. Get ready to focus and set those goals for yourself in the next chapter. Good luck!

# CONEY ISLAND

No fire or smoke showed on the outside of the building when the caravan of pumper and ladder trucks squeezed onto the block. The computer printout listed the reported location of the fire as the third floor of a 20-story apartment house, but the view from the street remained serene.

The morning's calm was suddenly shattered when a third-floor window let go with a loud pop that got everyone's attention. The fire had vented itself in backdraft fashion, shattering the window and allowing flames to race up the concrete facade.

An army of firefighters weighted down with heavy tools and high-pressure hoses filed into the building. My unit arrived first on the fire floor, and we made our way across that smoky hallway leading to the fire apartment. The metal apartment door was unlocked and hot to the touch as I hesitantly pushed it open.

Bang! I was struck with a searing blast of hot air that felt like I'd stuck my head in Mom's oven on Thanksgiving Day. The wave of heat catapulted all of us back 10 feet, fortunately into the protection of an enclosed stairwell. By now the engine company and their powerful hoses had arrived, our only weapons to slay the monster in apartment 3B.

A two-and-a-half-inch hose line used by the FDNY takes two or three strong men to operate and can deliver more than a thousand gallons of water in less than five minutes. Ruthlessly, feverishly, the hose team moved in and attacked. They kept low and close to the floor as they worked the powerful hose like a portable water cannon, bombarding the raging inferno, beating it back across the blackened corridor and into the apartment. Five minutes and a thousand gallons of water later, the monster was dead.

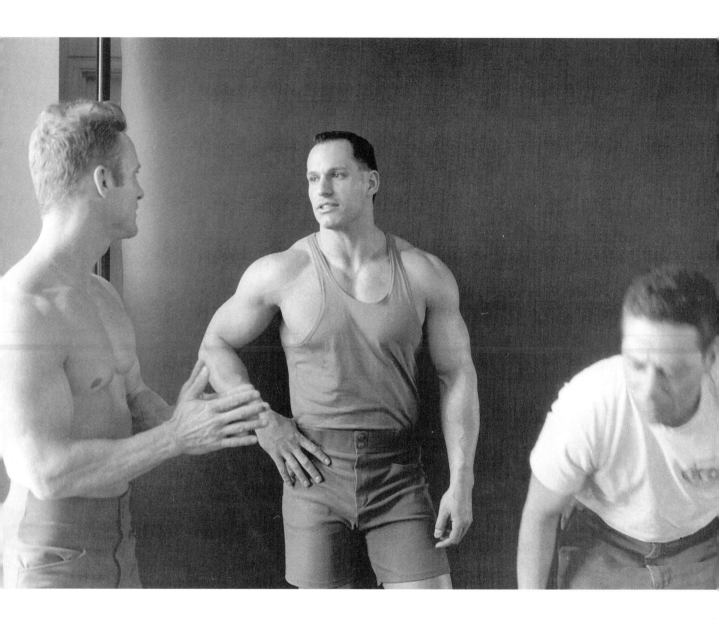

# CHAPTER TWO

# Mind over Matter

**A**s the mind thinks, the body follows. There is no way around that very simple concept. Your hopes, fears, desires, and the thoughts racing through your head right now all make up who and what you are. The truly powerful aspect of you is not your physical body but your mind.

At this point in your approach to fitness, you should have an idea *in your mind* of what you hope to achieve. You've peered down into your soul and decided that where you are now is *not* where you want to be. But where *do* you want to be? We can go no further until you uncover that vital piece of information. Be honest with yourself when you answer the following questions regarding your performance, appearance, and health.

### ▶ Performance

Do you want more physical strength, endurance and coordination?

Do you want to improve performance in a specific sport or activity?

### ▶ Appearance

Are you tired of the way you look and want to lose some body fat?

Do you want to put on muscle mass or just tone up and get leaner?

### ▶ Health

Has your health deteriorated to the point where you need to do something to improve it or maintain it?

Would you like to be stronger and more flexible and possibly prevent future injury?

Do you want or need more energy to make it through a long day?

The answers to these questions will help you form a clear picture in your mind of just where you want to be in terms of fitness. We'll call this your *ultimate fitness goal*, and it will be the driving force behind your workout program.

## SECTION 2.1    SETTING GOALS

Every day in life we set goals for ourselves that we can either live up to or fail miserably at. Not having clearly defined goals is one reason for failure. Some of my new clients aren't always sure exactly what they want from their exercise program. Before I begin training them, I insist they sit down with a pencil and paper and write down what they expect exercise to do for them, listing all possible goals and clearly defining them. We'll take it a step further and break down those goals into the following three categories:

1. *Ultimate goal.*   This is where you want to be—the finished product, so to speak. The answers to the questions at the beginning of this chapter will lead you to this in terms of performance, appearance and health. Your ultimate goal may not be achievable immediately, and there is no time frame for reaching it. It may take months or years, or you may never achieve this lofty prospect you've set for yourself, but that's okay. You'll come close enough to impact your life on every level. We'll see later in this chapter why you so sorely need to visualize this goal, like a magnet that you're irresistibly drawn to.

2. *Long-term goals.*   Here you set achievable goals within specific time frames ranging from three months to a year or more. Long-term goals can apply to every aspect of your training, from fat loss to how much weight you're lifting in a strength exercise to what pace you're able to keep during your cardio work. I suggest you set your long-term goals at three-month intervals and then reevaluate. By doing this you give your body a work order to perform the way you want it to within a specific time frame. This can be a very powerful process.

3. *Short-term goals.*   Goal setting in this category is the most immediate, and the goals should be the least challenging. Time frames range from one exercise within a workout to three months in the future. You want these goals to be totally achievable but still challenging. An example of a short-term goal would be setting the number of repetitions you'd like to complete during one set (increasing that number from workout to workout). Another example of an achievable short-term goal might be losing five pounds of fat in a month, or being able to maintain a faster pace in your aerobic workout.

You unconsciously set short-term goals for yourself every day, in every workout. When you get on the treadmill, for example, you have an idea of how long you're going to run or walk. That's a short-term goal. Take that one step further, and know *exactly how long and at what pace* you'll run. Monitor the effect by regular pulse checks and record this entire process (see Chapter 5), gradually increasing the duration and intensity levels as you progress.

Finally, don't underestimate the *rewards* aspect of goal setting. We're all like Pavlov's dogs in that we can be programmed to behave in a certain way. When you get through a really intense week of training, having achieved numerous short-term and maybe even long-term goals, give yourself the message loud and clear that you've succeeded. You will have your own idea of what a reward is, but it can range from a special dessert to scheduling an appointment for a professional massage. The greater the goal achieved, the greater the reward should be.

Figure 2.1 shows what a sample goals sheet might look like. Of course, your goals may be completely different, as they are a very individual choice.

## FIGURE 2.1    SAMPLE GOALS SHEET.

### Ultimate Goal

Performance
*Run the NYC marathon in less than three hours*

Appearance
*Weigh 175 pounds with 12% body fat*

Health
*Cholesterol level of below 150*

### Long-Term Goal

Performance
*Increase my cardio work to 30 minutes a session for three times a week in three months*

Appearance
*Fit into a size 6 by the year 2001*

Health
*Blood pressure reading of 120/70 in six months*

### Short-Term Goal

Performance
*Bench press 150 pounds for 10 repetitions next workout*

Appearance
*Lose five pounds in a month*

Health
*Eat no fried foods next week*

### NOTE

▷ You'll note that no time frames are listed under ultimate goals. If you have a set time frame in mind, list the goal as long term.

▷ As you can see, your goals can apply to every aspect of your training. Be creative. The only rule is to get in touch with what you *really want* out of your exercise and diet program.

▷ Goals change, so don't hesitate to list new goals as they occur, and cross off the ones you achieve.

## SECTION 2.2    HOCUS FOCUS

By now you've got a clear picture of where you want to be as your "finished product" (ultimate goal) and again at six months (long-term goal) or even at one month (short-term goal). The more clearly defined your goals are, the sharper your focus will become. In this section, you'll learn some techniques on how to maintain that focus.

## Unleash the Power of Your Mind

When you enter the gym, or before you head out for a run, think about what you are about to do. Take a few moments, even before your warmup, and get in touch with your body. Pay close attention to how you feel this day and what you would like to accomplish.

Any aches and pains? Do you feel energized or do you feel drained?

Bring your attention to your breathing.

## Energizing Breath

1. Sit quietly in a comfortable position, back and neck straight, mouth closed, while you breathe through your nose.
2. For the first few breaths, pay close attention to the flow without trying to affect it in any way.
3. Follow your inhalation as it flows through your nose and fills your lungs. Feel it energize your entire body.
4. Allow your abdomen to relax and expand *slightly*, pulling in even more air and energy.

5. Continue the in breath, allowing your chest to fill and expand as well. The total inhalation should be done for a count of 4.

6. Without pausing, begin your exhalation, allowing first the chest to empty, then your abdomen. Let all the day's tension, stress, and negativity flow from you along with your breath.

7. At the end of the exhalation phase, pull your stomach up and in, forcing more air out, increasing your lung capacity, and then inhale. The total exhalation should be done for a count of 8, or twice as long as the in breath.

Try to do 5 to 10 energizing breaths before each workout.

## Preworkout and Postworkout Meditation

Now continue to sit quietly and observe what's going on inside your body and your mind, as the two are so infinitely connected. Allow the image and qualities of your ultimate goal to permeate your entire being as you sit quietly and breathe deeply. Energize yourself with each in breath, and visualize this new you accomplishing all the goals you've laid out. See and feel yourself going through the upcoming workout effortlessly. Stay with this image as long as you can.

Get in touch with your body by learning to pay close attention to what it is telling you. Not every workout will be done at full intensity. You might be a little tired and fall short of your normal routine, or you might be in top form and go above and beyond it. Either way, consciously decide exactly how and what you'll be doing in this training session.

During your workout itself, observe the effect it's having on you. Try to put your mind into the muscles being worked and feel what's happening. After a while this will become second nature. At the end of your training session, again observe how your body feels.

Your cooldown is the time to bring your mind and body back from the intensity levels you maintained during the actual workout. Performing your flexibility movements at the end of your session is also a great way of maintaining that mind and body connection. When you're done stretching, sit quietly, breathe deeply, and again bring your mind back to your ultimate goal. Give yourself a little pat on the back and realize you're one step closer to achieving it.

## Priorities and Planning

We all have different things in life that are most important to us. Placing the proper amount of importance on your training and nutrition program is vital to your success. You've got to take it seriously, make a plan, and stick to it.

Know ahead of time each week when you're going to train and just what you're going to be training each session. Plan out your meals as well; don't just put food in your mouth without thinking (see Chapter 4). To the best of your ability, ensure that you'll have enough time to complete the required number of workouts to match your training goals. It's also a great idea to record all your exercise sessions, including informal comments about each one, using the blank workout chart given in Appendix C.

In the early nineties I worked with a firefighter who just couldn't say no. Bob was an exercise enthusiast who could never find the time to get in enough workouts to maintain the level of fitness he wanted. He led a very hectic life, mainly because he couldn't prioritize situations in his own life over what was important to the people around him. Bob eventually learned to say no and put his exercise and nutrition program above the wants and needs of everyone else in his life.

## Review

▶ Decide what your goals are as they relate to *performance, appearance,* and *health.*

▶ Record your *ultimate, long term,* and *short-term goals.*

▶ Reward yourself for achieving your goals.

▶ Use the *energizing breath* as a way to prepare your body for the upcoming workout and to release tension.

▶ Maintain your mental focus using the simple *meditation* presented.

▶ Pay close attention to what your body is telling you, and adjust your routine accordingly.

▶ Plan your training program and meals in advance.

▶ Set aside time each week to meet the demands of your exercise and nutrition program.

## BUSHWICK

All my years of training could have never prepared me for what happened on that frigid, windswept January night. Flames danced from the top-floor windows of the crumbling, vacant tenement building I stood in front of. Sprawled at my feet was a burning pile of black and yellow stripes. The stench of burnt flesh mixed with the smell of burning wood as I tried to focus on what was actually three firefighters who'd plunged from a third-floor window onto the cold, hard sidewalk. A sudden eruption of flame, fed by ferocious wind, had chased the trio to the front windows.

While perched on the narrow sill, flames licked violently at their backs. Ladders were frantically ripped from the trucks to attempt a rescue—but not fast enough. One by one—thud, thud, thud—their bodies collided with the unyielding concrete. Broken and lifeless they lay there, their blood pooling with the water being used to put out the smoldering fire on their charred backs.

Not one of them stirred. My frozen stare revealed the panic I was feeling as burning debris continued to rain down on the fallen heroes. A sea of firefighters swarmed the scene, and as if controlled by one mind, a dozen hands embraced the broken bodies and lifted them to shelter.

My radio crackled with a report of another firefighter trapped inside the building. My men and I realized what we had to do. I reached inside for every drop of strength and courage I could muster. We dragged our hose line into the inferno, and up the charred staircase, in search of another fallen brother.

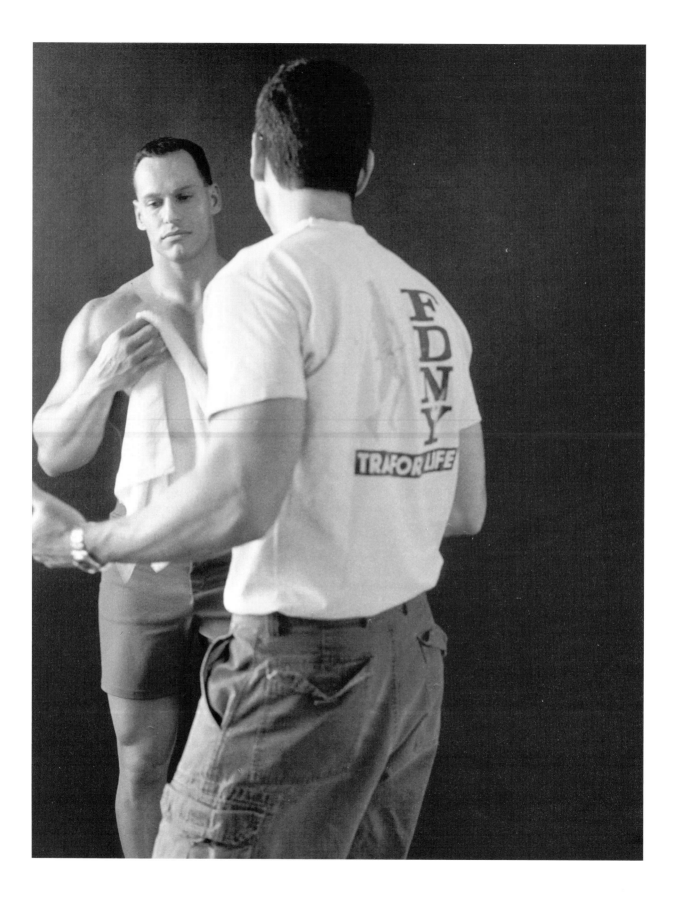

# CHAPTER THREE

# Principles of the Firefighter's Workout

**By now** you can tell that this is not just another how-to workout book, but rather a compilation of years of training experience, using proven formulas that will give you a healthy, strong, and lean body. These same principles were used successfully by many of New York City's firefighters and are still in use today. Remember, knowledge is power and knowing exactly *how* as well as *why* you're performing an exercise will make it that much more effective, saving you valuable time and effort and possibly needless injury.

The human body is an amazing machine in that the more you push it, the stronger it gets—up to a certain point. The body's ability to rise to the level of demand placed on it is known as the *adaptation response*, and we'll take advantage of that truly miraculous system as we attempt to push ourselves just a tiny bit more with each progressive workout.

In the pages that follow, I'll outline in a concise and simple format the theory and methodology behind the aerobic, strength, and flexibility training based on the adaptation response that has worked for New York's bravest.

We'll start with an overview of the *five components of fitness:*

1. *Muscular strength.* The strength of a muscle or muscle group is determined by how much resistance it can overcome in a single repetition. Those of us with a desire or need to create major increases in muscular strength (and mass) will achieve this through *strength training* (also known as *resistance training*) by lifting a heavy weight for only a few repetitions. The key to successful strength training is these low-rep sets done with high resistance. Having stronger muscles benefits all of us in some way, whether it be something as routine as pushing a heavy shopping cart around a supermarket or something crucial in nature, like the extreme demands of firefighting. More strength means that every task you encounter in everyday life is just plain easier.

2. *Muscular endurance.* Endurance of a particular muscle or muscle group is defined as how many times it can repeat a lift or hold a static position. Increases in endurance are achieved by working against light to moderate resistance for many repetitions. Some increase in muscle mass will be seen with endurance training, but most people will experience just a tightening or toning of the muscles worked. Muscular strength and endurance are

invariably intertwined, and any resistance training will increase both to a certain degree. We'll discuss weight and repetition ranges later in this chapter, but it's safe to assume that if you stay within the 8- to 15-repetition range, you'll achieve the maximum possible benefits of both strength and endurance training.

It's obvious how important muscular endurance is to a firefighter, but it can be equally important in your everyday life, as well. Every day you lift, reach, bend, and squat in your normal daily living. These are all minor demands on your endurance that are cumulative throughout the day.

Increases in muscular endurance gained through exercise keep us energized and help us to avoid that overly fatigued, run-down feeling we'd all love to forget. It can make daily activities a pleasure instead of a painful grind.

3. *Flexibility.* This is an often-neglected aspect of fitness that leads to imbalances in the body as well as injury. Technically, it is defined as the range of motion about a joint, but it also affects body awareness and posture. In simple terms, your level of flexibility is what limits how far you can bend or twist without pain or injury. Flexibility is most easily and safely achieved with static stretches and holds, in which you slowly bend into position until slight discomfort is felt and then hold that position for 15 to 30 seconds. This type of stretching produces a permanent elongation of muscle and connective tissue that enables you to move further and more freely without injury. If a highly flexible person were to take the same fall on a banana peel as a not-so-flexible person, chances are the more limber person would sustain less sprain- and strain-type injury to joints and connective tissue. The more elastic quality of the tissues enables his or her body to have more pliability and to give more before it tears or breaks down altogether.

4. *Cardiorespiratory endurance.* The ability to sustain muscle activity over time in relation to the heart-lung system defines cardiorespiratory endurance. The only way to achieve this is through an aerobic exercise that elevates the heart and breathing rates and is sustained for a specific period of time. While minor muscle building and toning will result from aerobic exercise, it's the most efficient way to burn fat. When you jog, for example, you are exercising aerobically, burning large amounts of stored body fat as well as maintaining the efficiency of the heart and lungs, increasing cardiorespiratory endurance. Running as a way to maintain cardio fitness has become very popular in the New York City fire department. Each year dozens of competitive firefighter races, for the benefit of various good causes, are held throughout the city, and hundreds of firefighters run in the annual New York City Marathon.

5. *Body composition.* This is the makeup of the body in terms of relative percentages of body fat to fat-free mass (muscle and bone). Considered by exercise physiologists to be a true measure of how fit you are, your ratio of body fat to muscle can be lowered through resistance and aerobic training and, to a certain degree, by flexibility training. This combination of training methods (or *cross training*) seems to work synergistically, with the effects of each method being multiplied by the proper application of the other, and the burning of body fat is pushed to its maximum rate. Years ago, it was common for firefighters to be either strength trainers or runners, without almost no thought given to flexibility. Today, the proper combination of these three types of exercise enables much quicker and more permanent results, changing body-fat-to-muscle ratios. Later, in Chapter 6, various methods of testing body composition and fitness will be discussed.

Now that we've laid out the components of fitness, let's break our training down into three categories that will be discussed in detail later in this chapter:

1. *Cardiovascular or aerobic.* Burns fat and increases the efficiency of the cardiovascular system. Cardio training is an essential ingredient in this program because it considers the health and vitality of its user. There is simply no better way to increase the efficiency and health of your heart and lungs than with cardiovascular or aerobic training. When you run, swim, or perform any of the example exercises listed, the increased demand for oxygen causes your heart to beat more rapidly in an effort to deliver the needed oxygen and other vital nutrients to starving muscle tissues. This increase in demand is met in the long term by a stronger, more efficient heart-lung system.

   *Examples:* Running, walking, swimming, Stair-Master, and cycling.

2. *Strength or resistance.* Builds muscular strength and endurance through increases in muscle mass and tone. Firefighters need to be strong. Operating heavy tools and hoses require tremendous amounts of both upper- and lower-body strength and endurance.

   Lifting heavy objects comes naturally to firefighters, but resistance training is beneficial for everyone as long as you remember that what is considered *heavy* is relative to each individual. Nevertheless, lifting a heavy object repeatedly will cause the muscles involved in completing the lift to become somewhat bigger and more toned. The idea is to perform the lift safely and most effectively to maximize results.

   *Examples:* Bench press and sprinting.

3. *Flexibility.* Increases the body's ability to move and bend without injury through an elongation of the muscles, tendons, and ligaments. This elongation is the result of temporarily stretching a muscle and its connective tissues to their limit and briefly holding—much as you'd stretch a rubber band, except that some of the stretch remains each time you engage in flexibility training.

   Increasing your body's ability to be elastic and to sustain any unwanted force is another benefit. In the fire service, where overextending yourself on a daily basis is almost unavoidable, being able to move freely and move further without injury affords a lot of protection. This also applies to anyone engaged in any type of training program.

   *Examples:* Hamstring step stretch and yoga.

## SECTION 3.1    CARDIOVASCULAR CONDITIONING

Nothing is more important to overall health and fitness than cardiovascular or aerobic training. There are many facets to total fitness, but cardiovascular or aerobic conditioning is a true measure of how efficiently your body works, uses oxygen, and burns fat. While it's true that running or bike riding will not reshape your body like strength training does, they will teach your body to be an efficient fat-burning machine. Aerobic conditioning can also give firefighters the edge they need when they're called on to operate under extreme conditions, thereby reducing their risk of a cardiovascular incident (heart attack or stroke) as well as enabling them to perform their jobs even better. A firefighter who has to make it up 10 or 15 flights of stairs to reach a trapped occupant will be better able to cope with the demands of the situation when his or her heart and lungs can sustain him or her during the arduous climb.

The human body will respond to the caloric demands of running or any other aerobic activity by burning lots of fat. The body uses fat, carbohydrate (stored as glucose or glycogen), and, to a lesser extent, protein as fuel (see Chapter 4 for more information). When you're training aerobically (when your heart is working at 60 to 90 percent of its maximum capacity), stored body fat becomes the major source of fuel being burned. At a heart rate that's less than 60 percent or greater than 90 percent of maximum, the body is not working aerobically, and will burn less fat but rather will use stored glucose as its primary energy supply. When we discuss strength training, we'll talk more about the subaerobic (less than 60 percent of maximum heart rate) and anaerobic (greater than 90 percent of maximum) aspects of the workout program.

Although it's inevitable (and even necessary) that you burn some sugar as well as fat, the goal is to burn more fat. Aerobic exercise achieves that goal. And, it not only burns fat while you're actually engaged in it, but teaches the body to be a more efficient fat burner on a 24-hour-a-day basis by building new fat-burning enzymes in response to the consistent demand (adaptation response) placed on it. If your aerobic workout is done properly (that is, if you elevate your heart rate to between 60 and 90 percent of its maximum capacity for at least 15 minutes) and consistently (three times a week or more), you'll teach your body to be a fat-burning machine even when you're not actually training. In other words, when you are sitting back on your living-room sofa watching a movie, munching on pretzels, you'll be burning fat!

## The Target Heart-Rate Zone

Monitoring your heart rate during exercise is a very simple method of ensuring that you're working aerobically and that you're burning the most fat you can. The idea, as mentioned, is to get your heart to beat at 60 percent to 90 percent of its capacity for a minimum of 15 minutes. Anything less than 60 percent is subaerobic and will not burn fat efficiently, while a heart rate greater than 90 percent of your maximum capacity is anaerobic and will tend to burn more carbohydrate (or glucose) than stored body fat. In order to calculate your *maximum heart rate* (MHR) safely, use the following formula:

220 − your age = your maximum heart rate

For example, a 40-year-old woman's estimated maximum heart rate would be:

220 (arbitrary number) − 40 (age)
= 180 (estimated MHR)
60 percent of 180 (multiply $180 \times 0.6$)
= 108 (low end)
90 percent of 180 (multiply $180 \times 0.9$)
= 160 (high end)

According to this formula, the estimated zone for a typical 40-year-old woman is between 108 and 160. This is the number of times per minute her heart will beat when her body is burning fat *most* efficiently. As a beginner, you'll achieve results at the low end of the zone (60 to 70 percent), and to be most effective this rate should be maintained for at least 15 minutes, with a goal of 20 or 30 minutes. Using the *target heart-rate zone* as a tool in your fitness toolbox will become second nature after a while, so don't get discouraged if it seems a little complicated at first. Using a calculator will simplify matters for those who are mathematically impaired (myself included).

## Methods of Monitoring Heart Rate

Determining your heart rate usually requires you to stop whatever activity you're engaged in and take a *quick pulse check*. The pulse can be felt at either the carotid artery in the neck or the radial artery at the wrist.

### Carotid Artery (Neck)

Using the index and middle fingers of your right hand, gently feel for the notch between the muscles in your neck and your windpipe on the right side of your neck *without reaching across to the other side.*

Do a six-second pulse check and multiply by 10. Any longer than six seconds will allow the heart to slow down and will give you an inaccurate reading. Note your results.

### Radial Artery (Wrist)

Using the same two fingers (index and middle) of the right hand, gently feel for the notch on the underside of the left wrist, just above the thumb. Do the same six-second pulse check and multiply by 10.

### Heart-Rate Monitor

Another option is a heart-rate monitor, which is available at your local sporting goods store for less than $100. This is a very simple piece of equipment that lets you keep a constant eye on your heart rate without having to pause to do pulse checks. One size fits all, and it conveniently straps to your wrist like a watch.

### Talk Test Method

Unfortunately, the 220-minus-your-age formula doesn't apply to everyone, as some people's MHRs are just higher than others'. Unlike your resting heart rate, which can be lowered through exercise, your MHR cannot be affected. To accurately determine your MHR, you must engage in a type of physical activity, such as sprinting, that elevates your heart rate to its maximum. This can be very risky for some individuals and is not recommend unless you're quite fit to begin with. A safer alternative would be to use the talk test.

The *talk test method* relies on your *breathing rate* rather than your heart rate. The following list can be used to safely determine if you're exercising aerobically or not:

| | |
|---|---|
| *Below aerobic* | Breathing comfortably, talking easily |
| *Aerobic* | Breathing deeply, talking haltingly |
| *Anaerobic* | Wheezing, unable to string three words together |

# Warming Up and Cooling Down

The time in the target heart-rate zone doesn't include the warmup or cooldown and those will have to be added into your total workout time as well. Warming up and cooling down can simply be five minutes of a lighter version of the same activity. For example, walking serves as a perfect warmup as well as a cooldown for running.

# Choosing the Right Aerobic Exercise for You

With all the new exercise equipment and infomercials out there, making a decision on your mode of aerobic conditioning could be quite confusing. A lot also depends on your level of fitness. While it might be necessary for a fit person to run to get into the aerobic zone, an unfit person could achieve the same result by walking. In order for a movement to be aerobic, a few basic rules apply:

► It uses the larger muscles of the legs and buttocks.
► It is sustained for at least 15 minutes.
► It puts the exerciser into the target heart-rate zone (as previously explained).

**COMMON AEROBIC EXERCISES**
Running
Jogging
Walking
Bicycle riding
Stationary bicycle riding
Jumping rope
Cross-country skiing
Swimming

The type or mode of cardiovascular training you choose is not as important as getting yourself into the zone during the activity. Whether it's running outdoors or riding a stationary bike, the fastest way to burn a lot of fat is to ensure you're getting into the target heart-rate zone by using your pulse or breathing rate as a guide.

Whatever method you choose, I encourage you to mix things up and change your routine frequently. Working with the variables of cardiovascular training, the combinations are endless.

# Variables of Aerobic Conditioning

The variables of aerobic conditioning include *modality*, *duration*, *frequency*, and *intensity*.

## Modality (How)

This refers to the actual type of exercise you choose, whether it's running, walking, or riding a stationary bicycle. This is usually a personal preference, although some movements are more efficient than others in elevating your heart rate. The more muscles involved in the movement, the more efficient it will be in getting you into the target heart-rate zone. Some people like running outdoors, while others love the solitude of their treadmills. I encourage you to change your mode of cardio exercise frequently to avoid boredom and possible overuse injuries that can be sustained by repeating the same movements over and over.

## Duration (How Long)

This refers to the length of time spent in the training session. Any aerobic workout should be preceded by five minutes of a lighter version of the same movement. This warmup slowly allows the muscles to lubricate themselves and prepare for a heavier workload. It also allows for the gradual increase in pulse rate and blood pressure, a must for anyone with hypertension or heart disease. Just as important as the warmup is the cooldown, which can also be a milder version of the same movement. It brings the body slowly through the changes of an intense workout to its normal resting state. Cooldowns should be long enough to allow the pulse and breathing rate to get to near normal, usually about five minutes. Duration is the length of time spent in the target heart-rate zone, between the warmup and the cooldown. The minimum time spent here should be between 15 and 30 minutes for an effective fat-burning aerobic session.

## Frequency (How Often)

This refers to the number of times per week (or per any specific length of time) you engage in cardiovascular training. Your frequency level can be influenced by many other factors, including the duration and intensity of your workouts. Another major consideration will be whether or not you're strength training simultaneously (cross training). If the major thrust of your entire workout routine is to build muscle mass versus burning fat, the frequency of your aerobic workouts should be less than if the major thrust is for fat loss. I recommend a minimum of two or three times a week for exercisers who are serious strength trainers and up to six times a week for those whose greatest interest is in getting lean. Your typical weekend warrior might be happy just to tone up, develop more strength, speed, and coordination, and not worry about a few extra pounds while only running twice a week. Someone substantially overweight might be more concerned with fat burning and could schedule up to six aerobic workouts weekly.

## Intensity (How Hard)

When it applies to aerobic conditioning, *intensity* refers to your heart or breathing rate. To be in the target heart-rate zone you need to working at 60 to 90 percent of your maximum heart rate. Training at the high end without exceeding it will give fastest results. Training too intensely and raising your heart rate above 90 percent of its maximum capacity will cause the exercise to become anaerobic, and fat burning will greatly diminish. The greater your intensity, the more rest you'll need between workouts. While a gentle walk at 65 percent of your maximum capacity can probably be repeated every day, for most individuals, especially beginners, a run at 85 percent will require a day of rest in between repetitions. You can see how increasing intensity levels can get you fit while you work out less often, a major plus for anyone with a limited amount of time to invest in their workout program. Personally, in my own routine, I'd rather keep intensity levels high, but you might prefer slightly less intense and longer workouts. The decision will ultimately be yours to make.

# Cardiovascular Training General Guidelines

▶ Pick an exercise you like, suited to your level of fitness; it can be changed as frequently as you wish. Change the mode of exercise as often as you like. Besides being a great way to avoid boredom, this also helps to eliminate overuse injuries.

▶ Select proper footwear to match your activity. For example, don't wear basketball shoes to run.

▶ Always warm up, cool down, and stretch out (see the Flexibility Training section of this chapter).

▶ Beginners should *always* start slowly and increase their duration, frequency, and/or intensity levels gradually, avoiding overuse injuries and allowing the adaptation response to take effect.

▶ Ensure that you're in the target heart-rate zone by monitoring your pulse or breathing rate and using the formulas given in this chapter. Ensure that you're in the zone for at least 15 minutes. Working at the high end of the zone (near 90 percent of your MHR) will reduce the length of time of your training session while producing dramatic results, but progress can still achieved at the low end.

▶ Repeat your cardio workout anywhere from two to six times per week, depending on your fitness goals. If the main thrust of your entire routine is to burn fat, repeat your aerobic workouts more often.

▶ Record your training sessions as outlined in Chapter 5.

▶ Integrate your cardiovascular training with your strength and flexibility training by using the workout routines that apply to you, as presented in Chapter 5.

▶ If you're too out of shape to do anything else, just walk. Gradually increase the length and intensity of your walks, and be sure to do pulse checks at various intervals to determine where you are in relation to the target heart-rate zone.

▶ Anyone embarking upon an exercise program is advised to seek the advice of a health care professional and get a complete physical exam before beginning.

## SECTION 3.2   STRENGTH TRAINING

Nothing affects your physical appearance as much as strength training. You can run until the cows come home, but it won't reshape or sculpt your body unless you add some muscle-building exercises into your routine. This book isn't about becoming a body builder. It is about getting stronger and putting on lean muscle mass while losing body fat. As a New York City firefighter, being strong meant the physical demands of the job seemed easier. Strength or resistance training is the safest and most efficient way to get toned, lean, and strong. The human body is comprised of more than 200 bones, more than 600 muscles and interconnecting tendons and ligaments, all of which are affected by resistance training. That's right—over a period of time, bones respond to the demand placed upon them just as muscles and tendons do, by becoming thicker and denser. This is great news, especially for women, who have a tendency to lose bone mass as they get older. Strength training done properly, combined with a healthy lifestyle that includes a balanced diet, can interfere with this process of bone loss.

At one point I trained a couple in their midsixties, both avid exercise enthusiasts and both concerned about loss of body mass, especially bone loss. To their credit, when they came to me they'd already been training for years, and in addition to weight training they were both into a very aggressive boxing-type workout, in which most of the cardio work was in upper-body punches and working with a heavy bag. They looked and moved 15 years younger than their age and were both successful in maintaining as much lean mass as possible.

## Fat-Burning Factories

Muscle needs energy (calories) to function. Simply stated, the more muscle you can pack onto your frame, the more calories you'll burn just standing still. Muscle cells are little fat-burning factories that require some sugar and a lot of fat for fuel. If you can put on some lean muscle mass, you'll have the added benefit of burning more fat while your body is at rest. Strength training is an anaerobic exercise—meaning that while the exercise is being performed, the primary source of fuel for the muscles involved is glucose (sugar). So now you're thinking, "How am I going to burn fat lifting weights?" The answer is very simple, because the recovery from strength training (the time you spend resting after the workout is done) is aerobic. So while your body is recuperating after an intense training session, it's also burning fat. Again, the intensity level is the key. Of course, every movement is performed

within the limits of proper form and safety. Intensity doesn't necessarily mean an increase in the amount of weight lifted. There are many ways to create intensity in a workout, and I will explain them later in this chapter, as well as in Chapter 5.

## A Special Word to Women

Don't be afraid to lift weights. When it comes to sculpting the body, strength training gives you the most bang for your buck. Simply do the routines as they're outlined in Chapter 5. Combine this training with a balanced, low-fat diet. When you're satisfied with the level of fitness you've achieved, simply shift to a *maintenance program* (Chapter 5, Routine 4). If you neglect the strength aspect of your training, you simply won't be able to reshape your body. As an added benefit, you'll find that the more muscle you carry on your frame, the more fat is burned when you're *not* exercising, so you'll actually be able to eat more without getting fatter.

## Strength Training Overview

Nowhere is the adaptation response more evident than in strength training. A gradual increase in the resistance means a gradual improvement in the body's ability to handle it. The key here is *gradual* increase, because if you go beyond the body's ability to repair itself, injury will occur.

### First Things First

Warm up the entire body first. No matter what workout routine you're doing this day, start with 5 or 10 minutes of getting yourself warmed up. This can be a brisk walk on a treadmill or outdoors as well as a quick ride on a stationary bike. This general warmup is in addition to the first set of each exercise that's done with a very light weight for 20 repetitions (*specific warmup*).

## Big Muscles First

In Chapter 5, actual routines are charted, but if you analyze them, the larger muscles are always trained first. When you strength train for your legs, chest, and back (the three largest muscle groups), almost a third of the body's muscle is trained simultaneously. Major lifts such as this have the most beneficial effect when performed on muscles that are adequately warmed up but still fresh and strong, not prefatigued by minor lifts. In this way, the greatest amount of resistance can be overcome, resulting in the greatest muscle growth. Here's the priority order of the muscle groups:

1. Legs
2. Chest
3. Back
4. Shoulders
5. Arms
6. Core

See Appendix B for anatomical charts and details.

## Strength Versus Endurance— Deciding How Much to Lift

Performing sets with very low repetitions (fewer than eight) is not the fastest way to a toned, muscular body but will mostly result in the kind of muscular growth associated with power lifting. On the other hand, doing more than 15 or 20 reps does little in building any real mass but will result in toned (albeit not large) muscles. The recommended range is 8 to 15 reps on each set except for the warmup set, which should be 20. You must choose a weight that will allow you to hit at least muscle fatigue in that 8- to 15-rep range. *Muscle fatigue*, as defined in Appendix A, refers to the point in the exercise where you begin to experience some local discomfort and possible weakness in the muscle or muscle group being worked. Muscle failure implies that the muscle being worked absolutely cannot do another repetition without abandoning proper form (cheating) or bringing other muscles into play. In other words, at muscle fatigue you begin to feel some pain in the muscle being worked; at muscle failure the muscle or group being worked cannot do another rep.

As your body gets stronger, you must increase the amount of resistance you're working against. A simple way to ensure progress is to set up a system for yourself in which you add weight when a certain number of repetitions are reached.

*Example:* Lisa started doing bench presses with 10-pound dumbbells. On her first day, she was able to do *12 reps* to muscle fatigue. In two weeks' time, she found she could do *15 reps* with the same weight. At that point, she increased her resistance to *12-pound* dumbbells, and when she can do that 15 times while still maintaining proper form, she will increase it again.

## How Many Sets

Theoretically, if you can exhaust a muscle in one set, no more training of that muscle will be needed for maximum growth. The only problem with this system is the risk of injury at such a level of intensity. A more practical approach would be to do two, three, or four sets of slightly less intensity, with the first set acting as a warmup.

Resist the temptation to do too many sets. Ron, a firefighter I worked with, as well as trained occasionally, came to me with a get-fit-in-six-weeks program, wanting me to put him through 38 sets his first day. I flat-out refused and trained him as I would train any other client of his fitness level. The next workout, Ron made it to the gym on his own, doing almost 40 sets that day. He continued to do really long, too-many-set workouts for another week or two, until he was so dramatically run down that he got sick from overtraining (see Chapter 6 for more information on overtraining). If something works, more of it doesn't necessarily increase its effectiveness.

## Rest Between Sets

This is another variation that requires some discussion. For a beginner, a good rule of thumb is to rest for one to two minutes between each set unless otherwise indicated by some type of specific training protocol (for example, circuit training—Chapter 5, Routine 3). Less rest between sets tends to build more muscle endurance, while strength is enhanced with a longer rest between each set, allowing the muscle or muscle group to recover completely.

## Not All Positive

Every strength-training exercise will have two phases. In phase 1, the positive phase, the weight or resistance is *lifted* against gravity. This is the exhalation phase; it should be performed at a slow, controlled count of 2. In phase 2, the negative phase, the weight or resistance is controlled as it's *lowered* against gravity. This is done on inhalation to a slow count of 4, or twice as long as the positive phase. Some exercise physiologists feel that more muscle building actually occurs in the negative phase of the movement. As you become more advanced in your strength training, pay closer attention to proper form in the negative phase of each repetition as a way to accelerate muscle growth. As the weight or resistance is lowered against gravity, the muscle fibers perform a braking action, resulting in a very strong contraction. This can be used to your advantage in increasing the efficiency of your routine. See Chapter 5, Routine 6 for details.

## As Easy as ABC (Alignment, Breathing, and Control)

Maintaining proper form means following certain guidelines that apply to every set. This will increase the workload on the target muscle group, increasing

intensity with less weight. By increasing intensity in this fashion, you can still make incredible strength-training gains while reducing your risk of injuring joints and connective tissue due to overload.

### *Alignment*

Correctly align your body (working joints aligned with the axis of rotation) as per specific instructions for the exercise. Shoulders are kept back and down while your abdomen is held in and slightly up. The natural curve in your back is maintained, and your gaze is forward with the head straight. Each movement is outlined in detail in Chapter 5.

### *Breathing*

Exhale on the positive or up phase of the repetition, generally for a count of 2. Inhale on the negative or down phase for a count of 4, closing your mouth and breathing through the nose. Breathing is an important part of any training, because it not only serves to focus your mind into the movement but also replenishes vital oxygen.

### *Control*

Go through a full range of motion, slow and controlled, without cheating or using momentum to complete the lift. Keep your mind focused on the movement, making it as intense as possible.

Earlier in my career I trained two firefighters as different as night and day. The first guy loved adhering to perfect form, performing all his lifts with a moderate weight, in a slow and controlled manner, with proper breathing, alignment, and control on every lift. The second guy was the complete opposite, wanting to lift heavier weights with jerky, bouncing motions. No matter how hard I tried, I could not impress upon Firefighter Badform how much time and energy he was wasting lifting in this manner until I invited him to a session with his good twin, Firefighter Goodform. He was amazed at the muscle development Goodform had achieved in the same short months that he'd been training. He was able to put ego aside and begin with a moderate weight that enabled him to perform each movement properly, targeting the correct muscles and avoiding injury, putting himself on the road to success.

## Active Rest

This is a concept you can apply to some of the routines in Chapter 5. Basically, it allows you to back off your intensity, frequency, or duration on any given workout or in any given week. Sometimes your body just isn't up to a full-blown workout. You might be under the weather for whatever reason and just not be up to it. You can also incorporate this concept into your routine by scheduling one week every month as a *light week,* in which you back off on the amount of weight lifted or the duration and frequency of your workouts. Sort of a working vacation for your muscles.

## Delayed Muscle Soreness

Some soreness after intense physical exercise is considered normal and even a desired effect indicating the muscle did indeed work and will respond by getting stronger. As a matter of fact, by the time you feel this pain, you've already begun the healing process, and it should disappear in a day or two. You have to be able to distinguish between *delayed muscle soreness* (usually experienced 24 to 48 hours after exercise) and a muscle or joint injury. Normally, delayed muscle soreness (DMS) is located in the muscle itself, not in the associated joint. Activity of any kind invariably lessens the pain, and it usually peaks about 24 hours after the workout.

Pain associated with obvious deformities, swelling of the affected area, or skin discoloration, or any pain that doesn't go away in a few days, should be considered potentially dangerous. The injured area should be rested and examined by a physician before you return to your exercise program. Don't ignore pain of any kind—pay attention to it and to what causes it.

After training for a while, you'll be able to differentiate between DMS and pain resulting from an injury.

# Variables of Strength Training

The variables of strength training include *mode, duration, frequency,* and *intensity.*

## Mode (How)

This refers to the type of resistance equipment you use, ranging from the latest machines to simple dumbbells. As long as the muscle is placed under load it will respond, regardless of the source of resistance.

*Examples:* Different modes of strength training can be illustrated by a barbell squat, a health club machine chest press, or a dumbbell curl.

## Duration (How Long)

This refers to the length of time you spend in your strength-training session or the number of sets (volume) you do. Duration must be adjusted to allow for how hard (intensity) and how often (frequency) you train.

*Example:* Bill performed his strength-training program for a duration of 45 minutes twice a week, doing a full-body routine each time. He switched to a split routine four times a week for a duration of one hour.

## Intensity (How Hard)

This refers to how far past the point of *muscle fatigue* (the point in the set at which some discomfort or slight pain is felt in the muscle or group being worked) you are willing or able to go on the way to total *muscle failure* (the point in the set past muscle fatigue where doing another repetition is impossible without abandoning proper form). It's not necessary to work to failure on every set. On the contrary, a safer, more comfortable approach may be to lower your intensity slightly and increase the number of sets while the intensity from each set adds up. You have to find the balance that works for you, experimenting with the number of sets and how far past muscle fatigue you can comfortably go on a consistent basis and still make progress. Remember: Within the limits of safety, increasing intensity is the fastest way to increase lean muscle mass and produce dramatic results in the least amount of time. I recommend using a system of rating intensity on a scale of 1 to 5 and recording this with your workouts. You'll want to be between 2+ and 4 on most sets, reserving a level a 4+ or 5 for one possible final set on each exercise.

#### STRENGTH-TRAINING INTENSITY SCALE

| | |
|---|---|
| 1 | No workout |
| 2 | No muscle fatigue experienced during the lift |
| 3 | Minor muscle fatigue experienced on the last repetition |
| 4 | Major muscle fatigue felt on the last few repetitions |
| 5 | Total muscle failure, unable to perform one more repetition with proper form |
| + | Halfway to the next level |

### Frequency (How Often)

Refers to how often you repeat the workout or repeat the training of a specific muscle group. Muscles need rest to tone and develop, and the same muscle or group should not be worked two days in a row. I had a client, Helen, who insisted on working out on her own in between our intense strength-training sessions. The recommended frequency to retrain a muscle is from 48 to 96 hours for maximum effectiveness, and she was retraining the same muscle group only 24 hours later. The problem was corrected, and with Helen strength training only two or three times a week, she progressed rapidly. It's a relief to know that intense workouts need not be repeated every day to be effective.

# Strength Training General Guidelines

▶ Always warm up prior to and cool down and stretch out after your resistance workout.

▶ Whether you're training with sophisticated machines or simple dumbbells, proper form and adherence to the ABCs are essential to success and injury prevention.

▶ Select a weight or resistance level that coincides with your level of fitness and allows you to hit muscle fatigue at your desired repetition range (normally either 8 to 12 or 12 to 15, depending on your goals). Attempt to gradually increase the weight from workout to workout and, if called for in the specific routine, from set to set.

▶ Heavy weight lifted for low repetitions (fewer than 8) will build more strength and mass than a lighter weight lifted for a moderate number of repetitions (8 to 15), which will build more endurance while it tightens and tones. The first warmup set should generally be 20 reps.

▶ Rest between 48 and 96 hours before retraining the same muscle or muscle group. As a general rule, rest one to two minutes between each set unless contradicted by the protocol for a specific routine.

▶ Beginners should always start slowly, doing only as much as they can handle, and gradually increase resistance, taking advantage of the adaptation response.

▶ Vary your training program by changing exercises and routines every month or two.

▶ Record all your workouts (see Chapter 5) and use the 1-to-5 scale to rate your intensity.

▶ Ideally, your aerobic training and your strength training should be done on alternate days, but if you only have three days a week to work out, combine them. Be flexible in your scheduling.

▶ Pay attention to your body, and avoid overtraining by resting when necessary.

▶ Anyone embarking on an exercise program is advised to seek the advice of a health care professional and get a complete physical exam before beginning.

## SECTION 3.3    FLEXIBILITY TRAINING

Often an overlooked part of fitness, flexibility training figures prominently into the Firefighter's Workout. Chapter 1 showed what a powerful effect a properly supervised combined stretching and strengthening routine can have. A truly strong body must be limber or its strength is neither healthy nor functional. What you accomplish by stretching your tight muscles, tendons, and ligaments is *balance*. Balance from all the stresses and strains of everyday life as well as balance in training.

With flexibility training you're able to achieve a certain elasticity that is characteristic of youth. Your posture improves dramatically when tight chest and shoulder muscles don't pull forward. A limber body appears taller and more graceful. And as every firefighter who's participated in any stretching program knows, all those nasty sprains and strains are dramatically reduced. Just in case you're still not convinced, here are some more benefits of flexibility training:

▶ *Decreased risk of injury.*  Experts agree that by increasing your range of motion you reduce the likelihood of incurring injury. A flexible, bendable body simply won't break as easily.

▶ *Increased physical efficiency and performance.*  A flexible joint requires less energy to move through its full range of motion. Your body will be a more efficient machine.

▶ *Increased circulation.*  Greater blood flow to joint structures provides greater oxygen and nutrient transport where it's needed most, in the muscles and connective tissues.

▶ *Increased neuromuscular coordination.*  Studies have shown that nerve impulse velocity is improved with dynamic flex training, thereby improving performance in various athletic activities, such as a golf or tennis swing.

▶ *Improved muscular balance and posture awareness.*  Flexibility helps realign the body against the forces of gravity and bad posture, increasing your awareness of your body's position in space.

▶ *Decreased risk of lower-back pain.*  Flexibility of the lumbar, pelvis, hamstring, and hip flexors is crucial in reducing stress to the lumbar spine. When these muscles are too tight, they pull on the pelvis, causing an unnatural arch in the spine and resulting in pain and muscle weakness.

▶ *Reduced stress.*  Stretching promotes physical and mental relaxation associated with proper breathing techniques and yoga exercises.

*Flexibility* is defined as a joint's ability to move freely in every direction or, more specifically, through a full and normal range of motion. There are a number of factors that can limit joint mobility, including the following:

▶ *Structure of the joint.*  This varies from person to person, based on the shape of the bones and the length and attachment points of the tendons and ligaments.

▶ *Genetic inheritance.*  A certain built-in elasticity passed down from generation to generation; this will also vary from person to person.

▶ *Connective tissue elasticity within muscles, tendons, ligaments, or skin.* The soft tissue of your body naturally maintains a certain level of elasticity. The combined effect of all soft-tissue stiffness is what limits flexibility.

▶ *Opposing muscle group.* Each muscle group is paired with another muscle group that performs its exact opposite motion. For example, while the biceps flexes the forearm into a 90-degree angle, the triceps extends it to a straight-arm position from a 90 degree angle. The biceps and triceps are opposing muscle groups, and if one is too overdeveloped it will limit the flexibility of the opposite group.

▶ *Neuromuscular coordination.* Sometimes referred to as *hand-eye coordination,* this is the body's ability to send signals to working muscles in the blink of an eye (or even faster) in order to compensate for changes in the immediate environment. Those individuals with higher levels of neuromuscular coordination can usually achieve greater flexibility.

Flexibility training minimizes these factors and helps to balance muscle groups that might otherwise be overused during strength and cardiovascular training or even as the result of poor posture. Flexibility can be further broken down into static and dynamic flexibility:

▶ *Static flexibility.* This is *nonactive flexibility;* it involves the range of motion of a joint with little emphasis on speed.

▶ *Static (Passive) Stretch.* Low-force, gradual, controlled elongation of muscle and connective tissue through a full range of motion that produces a *permanent* stretch. Static stretching should usually be performed at some point during or at the end of an intense training program when body core temperatures are slightly elevated. This type of stretch promotes relaxation of muscle tissue and is held from 15 to 30 seconds for maximum effectiveness. An example of a static stretch is lying on your back while pulling both knees to your chest, holding for a specified period of time. This gentle elongation of the lower-back muscles produces a stretching effect that lasts after the position is released.

▶ *Dynamic flexibility.* This is *active flexibility;* it involves speed during physical activity. Strength, power, neuromuscular coordination, and tissue resistance are all factors in dynamic flexibility.

▶ *Ballistic (Dynamic) Stretch.* High-force, short-duration technique that employs rapid, uncontrolled bouncing or bobbing motions and produces a *temporary* stretch. Since many movements in sport and exercise are ballistic in nature, a dynamic stretching technique may be appropriate when specifically training for a sports activity but may be ignored in most exercise routines. Examples of ballistic stretches are a tennis player swiping at the first few balls or a baseball pitcher letting go of those first few pitches, able to increase speed and range of motion with each succeeding swing or throw.

## Flexibility Training General Guidelines

▶ The flexibility segment of your workout should be done when the body is warm, preferably at the end of either your aerobic or strength segments. However, stretching exercises can also be mixed in with strength movements to save time.

▶ As just stated, you cannot stretch a cold muscle—doing so will result in injury and will accomplish nothing.

▶ Static stretches should generally be held from 15 to 30 seconds. A sum total of 30 seconds is necessary to achieve any kind of permanent stretch.

▶ Breathe out when going into a stretch and inhale when coming out of it, using the breath as a way to go further into the movement.

▶ Never stretch to the point of feeling pain, just slight discomfort. If you experience pain, you're creating more tension and risking possible injury.

▶ Unlike strength-training or intense aerobic workouts, your flexibility segment can be repeated every day. Stretching has a healing effect on the body and does not require the same recuperation period as running or lifting weights.

▶ Vary the stretching exercises from day to day to ensure hitting all areas and relieving any boredom. If you follow the routines in Chapter 5, you'll find the exercises are somewhat varied.

▶ Again, beginners should start slowly and increase the length of time stretches are held or the number of sets per workout, taking advantage of that adaptation response. Another option might be to take it a step further and take a yoga class, which makes a great adjunct to the Firefighter's Workout.

▶ The flexibility segment of your workout can make a natural cooldown period for either an intense aerobic or strength-training session.

## SECTION 3.4 PUTTING IT ALL TOGETHER

The sign of a knowledgeable trainer is the ability to put all three aspects of training together in the right combination to achieve the results that the client is looking for. With the help of this book, you can be your own trainer and achieve the results you're looking for.

## How to Structure Your Workout Program

### Time

The first decision you'll have to make is how much time you are willing or able to devote to your program. The time factor involves two aspects, how many days a week you can train and how much time you can devote to each workout. Ideally, you'll be able to alternate strength- and cardiovascular-training sessions, which might require you to train four or five days a week. If you are able to devote only three days to your training sessions, you might have to opt for a program that combines the two workouts. Be flexible, and make your schedule work for you. With the Firefighter's Workout you can adjust your routine to fit you. When I lived in the city I used to train Mona, a busy professional and mother of four. She absolutely could not afford to train more than two days a week. She did her entire cardiovascular, strength, and flexi-

bility routine on both training days (which were never consecutive). Whenever she could, she'd squeeze in some physical activity between workouts, even if it was a simple game of catch in the backyard with one of her children. She made it work for her.

### Goals

We spoke a lot about goal setting in Chapter 2, but here we'll discuss it in relation to creating your program. Again, you've got to ask yourself certain questions about what you expect to get from your training program. Are you more interested in improving your health or in looking better? Do you want to trim down and lose fat or bulk up and gain muscle? These questions will decide what type of training you'll do most often and exactly how you'll train within each session.

### Certain Rules Apply

▶ Do more cardiovascular training and less strength training for fat loss and cardiovascular health.

▶ Use a light resistance and high repetitions (more than 15) to increase endurance and muscle tone.

▶ Use a heavy resistance and low repetitions (less than eight) to increase strength and muscle mass.

▶ A moderate resistance that allows you to complete 8 to 15 reps is ideal as it accomplishes a little of both endurance and strength gains.

▶ Determine how much weight you should lift in each set by setting the ideal number of repetitions to be completed that coincides with your individual goals.

# Equipment

A muscle doesn't know if it's working against a $5,000 health club machine or a $5 dumbbell. Resistance is resistance, but you'll still need a few items to start your training. Most firehouses in New York City are equipped with very simple gyms, not very fancy equipment, but they all get the job done.

## Bare Essentials

▶ *Dumbbells ranging from 5 to 15 pounds or more (or adjustable dumbbells).* This will form the core of your home gym. An absolute must.
▶ *Small bench (or workout step that can serve as a bench).* Many exercises require either sitting or lying on a bench.
▶ *Exercise mat.* A very simple but useful piece of equipment that enables you to do many floor moves safely and without rug burn.
▶ *Good shoes to match your activity (running, walking, or cross training).* This item cannot be overemphasized, especially if you're a runner. Improper shoes can lead to long-lasting overuse injuries. This can easily be avoided—always purchase the right shoes for your activity.

These items can be stored in a corner of a bedroom or slid under a bed, and they can all be purchased at your local sporting goods store for a little over $100.

## Optional Extra Equipment

▶ *Resistance tubing or resistance bands.* These make an excellent substitute for weights, and their portability makes them excellent for traveling.
▶ *Adjustable bench (flat, inclined, and upright).* This enables more advanced moves with heavier weights.

▶ *Barbell and sufficient weights for your level of fitness.* These enable more advanced moves with heavier weights.
▶ *Treadmill or stationary bicycle.* These make a great addition to any indoor gym.

# Functional Fitness

When it comes to fitness, most of us think in terms of improved health and appearance, whereas the goals of the competitive athlete or firefighter can be more performance oriented. Certain movements, whether they are aerobic or anaerobic exercises, more closely mimic normal human movement. For example, squats and/or lunges (Chapter 5) work not only the quadriceps, hamstring, and gluteus (buttock) muscles but also important stabilizer muscles of the lower torso, while at the same time requiring the maintainence of *balance*. These functional movements not only increase performance in everyday life, but also help to eliminate problems caused by poor body awareness. Exercises that isolate a specific joint and act on one muscle still have a place in your routine. Beginners and individuals developing hard-to-reach areas or recovering from an injury will find isolated movements useful. When training firefighters, I like to use as many functional exercises as possible, better preparing them for the rigors of the job.

| FUNCTIONAL EXERCISES | ISOLATED EXERCISES |
|---|---|
| Squat | Leg extension |
| Lunge | Leg curl |
| Bench press | Fly |
| Standing curl | Seated dumbbell curl |
| Shoulder press | Lateral raise |
| Row | Pull-down |
| Sit-up | Leg raises |
| Dips | Lying triceps press |
| Push-up | Pec deck |
| Running | Stationary bicycling |

## A Plan

▶ Exercise at least three times a week and include some cardiovascular, strength, and flexibility training.

▶ Eat a balanced diet that includes a lot of fresh fruits and vegetables with the proper balance of carbohydrates, protein, and fat (Chapter 4).

▶ Drink eight glasses of water per day (Chapter 4).

▶ Don't smoke and drink alcohol only in moderation.

▶ Give your body the rest it needs by sleeping six to eight hours nightly, depending on your individual needs.

## Integration

If your aerobic work is to be done with your strength training, I recommend it be done afterward as it tends to take away from the intensity of your strength workouts. Otherwise, do your strength and cardiovascular work on alternate days. Never perform the same strength exercises two days in a row, and beginners shouldn't engage in intense aerobic training without a day of rest between workouts. Make sure you completely rest at least one day a week no matter what type of training you're engaged in. Flexibility training is the exception to this rule; it can be done every day due to its gentle effect on the body.

Chapter 5 contains training programs and methods already charted that integrate strength, cardiovascular, and flexibility training. Just pick the routine that matches your time constraints and fitness goals, and get ready to have the body of your life!

## CHOW'S NOT ON

January is always frigid in New York City, and that night was no exception. The evening meal was being methodically dished, but as fate would have it, the alarm rang out just as the mashed potatoes hit my plate.

The computer told us smoke was coming from the windows of a vacant building on a familiar block notorious for vacant-building fires. As I boarded the truck I geared myself up for what I knew I'd be hearing any moment from the Brooklyn fire dispatcher, "Brooklyn to Engine 22." "Go ahead Brooklyn," I answered. "We're getting multiple phone calls on this one, it sounds like you'll be going to work."

As we screeched around the corner, I saw fire blowing out of three front windows of a decrepit old vacant building that stood in the middle of the block like the last lonely old soldier finally ready to die. My crew and I had a different idea. Going into our normal routine, we raced to get a hose line to the seat of this inferno, and in about 10 minutes the fire was basically out, with some small hidden pockets remaining behind wall and ceiling plaster, fueled by the old, dry wooden studs.

The cold sneaked up on us once our adrenaline levels dwindled. I realized that my feet felt like blocks of ice. The firefighters on the hose line were drenched from wrestling with the high-pressure hose while a biting wind howled through the shell of the building. Standing there, watching them literally shivering in their boots, I heard the chief's voice crackle over my radio, "I'm going to leave you guys here to finish up, make sure you get all that hidden fire before you leave the scene." My stomach growled, and my body shook with cold, but all I managed to get out was "Ten-four, Chief."

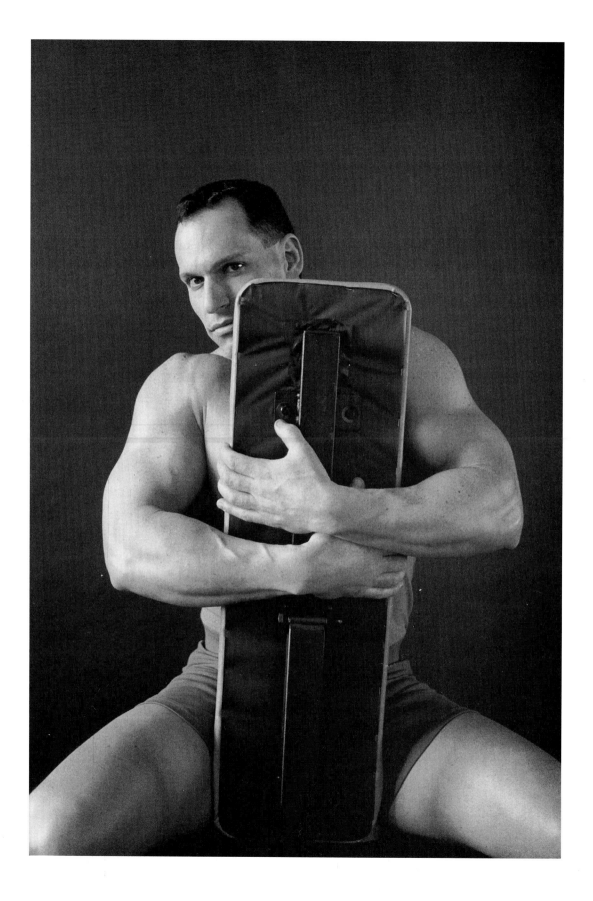

# Chow's On

**A**mericans are always on diets these days, and despite this we're getting fatter. Slim is in, yet as a society we remain mostly overweight. Health care costs continue to skyrocket as our crowded hospitals treat many obesity-related diseases such as atherosclerosis and adult-onset diabetes. As individuals, we need to take charge of this situation and do something about it. One of the things we can do is to stop trying to lose weight through unhealthy diets and take a sensible approach to losing excess body fat.

Fad diets that enjoy so much popularity today are usually deficient in vital nutrients (see Section 4.2). This inhibits your ability to add or even maintain lean muscle mass. Even if these diets do provide some temporary weight loss, most of it will invariably come from lost muscle. Any diet that results in a loss of lean muscle mass is not going to work. Many women fall into this trap of working out and not eating enough to sustain and support those intense workouts. Men (especially firefighters) will generally overeat, and their problem stems from too many calories.

Your body is made up of a certain percentage of fat and a certain percentage of lean muscle mass. A healthy body-fat percentage for an adult male is about 15 percent, and for an adult female it's about 22 percent. I've trained clients with body-fat percentages ranging from as low as 8 percent to as high as over 30 percent. Monitoring not only your body weight but also your body fat will assist you in keeping your exercise and nutrition program on course. There are many methods to determine your body-fat percentage, including the expensive but very accurate water-immersion method and the slightly less accurate but more practical skin-fold measurement method, just to name two. A skin-fold caliper with an instruction booklet and associated charts can easily be purchased at select sporting goods or health food stores. See Chapter 6 for more details on this convenient and inexpensive method of body-fat assessment.

Fat is burned strictly by muscle tissue. About 30 percent of a healthy woman's body and about 40 percent of a healthy man's body is made up of muscle tissue, but that muscle burns almost 100 percent of the fat. Increase the muscle-to-fat ratio and you'll burn more fat, it's that simple.

What you need is a simple program that will assist you in losing fat without sacrificing lean muscle mass. It's got to deliver a balanced, highly nutritious, relatively low calorie diet that's easy to follow.

The next section of this chapter presents the *four-food-group system*, a simple yet effective way to manage your food intake while assuring an adequate consumption of all the vital nutrients necessary for the growth and development of a lean, healthy body. Following this system will take the guesswork out of determining how much and exactly what you need to eat on a daily basis.

## SECTION 4.1 THE FOUR FOOD GROUPS

The key to any healthy diet is variety. No one food can provide all the nutrients your body needs. Categorizing all foods according to their main ingredients, we arrive at the four-food-group system:

| Group 1 | Meat, fish, eggs, beans, and nuts | Contain large amounts of protein, niacin, and iron |
| Group 2 | Milk, cheese, and yogurt | Contain large amounts of protein, riboflavin, and calcium |
| Group 3 | Grains, bread, and cereals | Contain large amounts of carbohydrate, fiber, and B vitamins |
| Group 4 | Vegetables and fruits | Contain large amounts of carbohydrate, fiber, and vitamins A and C |

You'll note that fat and sugar are not listed in any food group. We'll treat them as nonfoods, but you'll still get plenty of fat and sugar mixed in with food from Groups 1 to 4.

**FATS AND SUGARS TO AVOID**

| | |
|---|---|
| Butter | Fried foods |
| Oil | Salad dressings |
| Margarine | Sour cream |
| Mayonnaise | Table sugar |

**LOW-FAT ALTERNATIVES**

| | |
|---|---|
| Nonfat yogurt | Skinless chicken breast |
| Buttermilk | Water-packed tuna |
| Skim milk | Split peas |
| Skim cottage cheese | Lentils |

## Nutrient Density

Some foods have a very low nutrient-to-calorie ratio, meaning you've got to consume a lot of calories just to get a few nutrients. Usually, the more processed and refined a food is the fewer nutrients per calorie it contains. Do your best to avoid overprocessed food. Many foods that form the average American diet tend to be nutrient deficient compared to the calorie wallop they deliver. Examples of such foods are the ever-popular french fries and various cakes, donuts, and cookies. Most fresh fruits and vegetables are very nutrient dense foods, especially in their raw state with no garnishes added.

## FIGURE 4.1   THE FOUR-FOOD-GROUP SYSTEM.

| Meat group | Milk group | Grain group | Vegetable and fruit group |
|---|---|---|---|
| *(2–3 servings daily)* | *(2–3 servings daily)* | *(at least 4 servings daily)* | *(at least 4 servings daily)* |
| Beans | Nonfat yogurt | Brown rice | Whole vegetables |
| Fish | Skim milk | Whole-wheat bread | Whole fruits |
| Chicken | Low-fat cheese | Oatmeal | Fruit juices |
| Beef | Yogurt | Whole-grain cereal | Vegetable juices |
| Eggs | Milk | Pasta | Dried fruits |
| Pork | | White bread | |
| | | White rice | |

## TABLE 4.1   SERVINGS MADE SIMPLE

| DAILY SERVINGS | GROUP | SERVING SIZE |
|---|---|---|
| 2–3 | Milk or yogurt | 1 cup |
| | Cheese | 1½ ounces |
| | Cottage cheese | 2 cups |
| 2–3 | Meat | 2 to 3 ounces (meat, poultry, or fish) |
| | Beans | 1½ cups |
| | Eggs | 2 |
| | Peanut butter | 2 tablespoons |
| | Nuts | ½ to 1 cup |
| At least 4 | Vegetables | ½ cup raw or cooked vegetables |
| | Fruits | 1 cup greens |
| | | ½ cup vegetable juice |
| | | ¼ cup dried fruit |
| | | ½ cup cooked fruit |
| | | ¾ cup fruit juice |
| | | 1 whole piece of fruit |
| At least 4 | Breads | 1 slice bread |
| | Cereal | 1 ounce ready-to-eat cereal |
| | Rice | ½ to ¾ cup cooked cereal, pasta, or rice |
| | Pasta | |
| Use sparingly | Fat | |
| | Oils | |
| | Sweets | |

## Guidelines

▶ Use the four-food-group chart in Figure 4.1 as a guide to assist you in your daily diet regimen.

▶ Start out with plenty of *breads, cereals, rice, pasta, vegetables, and fruits;* add two or three servings from the *meat group* (Group 1) and two or three servings from the *milk group* (Group 2). See Table 4.1 for serving sizes.

▶ Each food group provides some but not all the nutrients you need. Every effort should be made to spread the servings out over six small meals daily.

▶ Remember to use moderation when choosing from the "nonfood group," fat and sugar.

▶ The foods at the top of each list in the chart represent the lowest fat and calorie counts within that group.

| TABLE 4.2 | PROTEIN CHART | |
|---|---|---|
| **FOOD** | **SERVING SIZE** | **GRAMS PROTEIN** |
| Chicken breast | 3½ ounces | 30 |
| Tuna | 3½ ounces | 28 |
| Lean red meat | 3½ ounces | 25 |
| Egg or egg white | 1 egg | 8 |
| Cheese | 1 ounce | 8 |
| Milk or skim milk | 1 cup | 8 |
| Yogurt | 1 cup | 8 |
| Peanut butter | 1 tablespoon | 4 |
| Pasta | 1 cup | 4 |

Use the protein chart in Table 4.2 to assist you in regulating your protein intake, which is vital to the building of lean muscle mass.

## SECTION 4.2    SIX MAJOR CLASSES OF NUTRIENTS

### Protein

Protein is comprised of amino acids that build and repair body tissue, including bones, muscles, tendons, and ligaments. Protein is a major component of enzymes, hormones, and antibodies. When you work out you raise your daily requirement of protein.

### Recommended Daily Intake

One gram per kilogram of body weight or 12 to 20 percent of total caloric intake for average adults; 1.2 to 1.7 grams per kilogram of body weight for resistance or endurance athletes. Convert pounds to kilograms by dividing pounds by 2.2.

*Example:* A 150-pound average adult weighs 68 kilograms:

$$\frac{150 \text{ pounds}}{2.2} = 68 \text{ kilograms}$$

This translates into a daily intake of 68 grams of protein for the average adult and 82 to 116 grams of protein for the resistance or endurance athlete.

One gram of protein contains 4 calories.

**COMMENT:** If adequate calories of carbohydrates are not eaten, the body breaks down protein and uses it as a primary source of energy at the expense of the creation and maintenance of lean muscle mass. Studies have shown that resistance and endurance athletes have an increased need for protein.

### High-Protein Foods

Examples include meat, poultry, fish, eggs, and dry beans.

# Carbohydrates

Carbohydrates are converted to *glycogen* and are a primary fuel for the body. Carbohydrates also aid the body in using fat more efficiently. The human body is unable to store a lot of carbohydrate; therefore, supplies must be replenished often through diet.

## Recommended Daily Intake

Four to six grams per kilogram of body weight, depending on *activity level*, or 55 to 65 percent of total caloric intake. Active adults should consume about 65 percent of their total calories in the form of carbohydrates.

Convert pounds to kilograms by dividing pounds by 2.2.

One gram of carbohydrate contains 4 calories.

**COMMENT:** It takes 24 hours after intense exercise before *muscle glycogen* (or sugar) is restored. Studies have shown that when carbohydrate consumption is delayed after exercise, muscle glycogen storage is reduced and recovery is impaired. If you're having trouble maintaining normal workout intensities, you may have low levels of stored muscle glycogen.

## High-Carbohydrate Foods

Examples include bread, cereal, rice, pasta, fruit, and vegetables.

# Fats

Fats or *lipids* are the body's chief form of stored energy; the body also uses fat for insulation and the protection of vital organs. Fat is the major source of fuel for light- to moderate-intensity exercise. Essential fatty acids are necessary for the proper functioning of cell membranes, skin, and hormones and for the transportation of fat-soluble vitamins.

## Recommended Daily Intake

Approximately 30 to 65 grams, depending on *caloric consumption*, or 20 to 30 percent of total caloric intake.

One gram of fat contains 9 calories (more than double that of carbohydrate and protein).

**COMMENT:** The human body stores anything it consumes in excess of what it needs in the form of fat. You need to recognize the many sources of hidden fats in foods and limit your daily fat intake. A low-fat, high-carbohydrate diet increases muscle glycogen and is an important step toward a lean, fit body.

## High-Fat Foods

Examples include oils, ice cream, cake, butter, margarine, mayonnaise, bacon, and fried chicken.

# Vitamins

**NOTE:** RDA = U.S. recommended daily allowance for adults and children over 4 years of age; mg = milligrams; mcg = micrograms; IU = international units.

**A (CAROTENE)**
RDA: 5,000 IU daily
Formation and maintenance of skin, hair, and mucus membranes; aids in seeing in dim light; bone and tooth growth
Found in yellow and orange fruits and vegetables and green leafy vegetables

**B₁ (THIAMINE)**
RDA: 1 mg daily
Helps in releasing energy from carbohydrates during normal metabolism, growth
Aids in maintaining muscle tone
Found in cereal, oatmeal, meat, rice, pasta, and whole grains

### B$_2$ (RIBOFLAVIN)

RDA: 1.7 mg daily

Helps in releasing energy from protein, fats, and carbohydrates during normal metabolism

Found in leafy vegetables, whole grains, meat, eggs, and milk

### B6 (PYRIDOXINE)

RDA: 2 mg daily

Builds body tissue and aids in the metabolism of protein

Found in poultry, fish, lean meat, dried beans, whole grains, prunes, and avocados

### B$_{12}$ (COBALAMIN)

RDA: 6 mcg daily

Aids in the development of cells and the nervous system and in the metabolism of protein and fats

Found in meat, milk, and fish

### BIOTIN

RDA: 0.3 mg daily

Aids in the metabolism of protein, fats, and carbohydrates

Found in cereal, grain products, legumes

### FOLIC ACID

RDA: 0.4 mg daily

Aids in red blood cell production and genetic material development

Found in green leafy vegetables, meat, beans, peas, and lentils

### NIACIN

RDA: 20 mg daily

Aids in the metabolism of protein, fats, and carbohydrates

Found in meat, fish, poultry, cereals, peanuts, potatoes, eggs, and dairy products

### PANTOTHENIC ACID

RDA: 10 mg daily

Releases energy from fats and carbohydrates

Found in lean meat, whole grains, legumes, fruits, and vegetables

### C (ASCORBIC ACID)

RDA: 60 mg daily

Essential for formation of bone, cartilage, muscles, and blood vessels; also helps in the maintenance of capillaries and gums

Found in citrus fruits, berries, and vegetables

### D

RDA: 400 IU daily

Aids in bone and tooth formation; also helps maintain the action of the heart and nervous system

Found in milk, sunlight, fish, and eggs

### E

RDA: 30 IU daily

Aids in the protection of blood cells, body tissue, and fatty acids

Found in multigrain cereals, nuts, wheat germ, vegetable oils, and green leafy vegetables

# Minerals

### CALCIUM

RDA: 1,000 mg daily

Formation of strong bones, teeth, and muscle tissue; also involved in the regulation of heartbeat, muscle action, and nerve function

Found in milk and milk products

### CHROMIUM

RDA: Not established

Glucose metabolism; increases the effectiveness of insulin

Found in corn oils, whole grain cereals, and brewer's yeast

**COPPER**

RDA: 2 mg daily

Formation of red blood cells; bone growth; works with vitamin C

Found in nuts, meat, and legumes

**IODINE**

RDA: 150 mcg daily

Component of the hormone thyroxine, which controls metabolism

Found in iodized salt and seafood

**MAGNESIUM**

RDA: Not established

Acid/alkaline balance; aids in the metabolism of carbohydrates, minerals, and sugar

Found in nuts, green vegetables, and whole grains

**PHOSPHORUS**

RDA: 1,000 mg daily

Important in bone development and protein, carbohydrate, and fat utilization

Found in meat, fish, poultry, eggs, and grains

**POTASSIUM**

RDA: Not established

Fluid balance; controls the activity of the heart muscle, kidneys, and nervous system

Found in lean meat, fruits, and vegetables

**SELENIUM**

RDA: 50 to 200 mcg daily (provisionally established RDA)

Protects body tissues against damage from radiation, pollution, and normal metabolic processing

Found in fish, organ meats, lean meats, and grains

**ZINC**

RDA: 15 mg daily

Aids in digestion, metabolism, development of the reproductive system, and healing

Found in lean meat, eggs, seafood, and whole grains

# Water

Water enables chemical reactions to take place. The body is comprised of 60 percent water. Water is essential for life because the body cannot store it or conserve it.

## Recommended Daily Intake

Three to four quarts for adults.

## A Word about Dehydration

Dehydration is a major concern for members of the fire service or for anyone who works out. Exercisers who allow their bodies to dehydrate will fatigue earlier and lose coordination. To avoid this problem, drink fluid before, during, and after a workout. If you rely on thirst as an indicator, you will replenish only about half the lost fluid. Don't wait until you're thirsty to drink, and don't stop once your thirst is quenched. At the scene of an alarm, firefighters don't have the luxury of taking a break and getting a drink until their assignment is complete, and by that time it may be too late.

Firefighters across the country have been trained to remain hydrated between alarms while performing other routine duties. Serious dehydration can lead to heat exhaustion and a life-threatening condition known as *heat stroke.* All of this can be easily avoided by consuming nature's most abundant resource, water.

## Sensible Guidelines for Fluid Replacement and Exercise:

➤ Consume one to two cups of water (8 to 16 ounces) at least one hour before the start of exercise. If possible, consume eight ounces of water 20 minutes before the start of exercise.

➤ Consume four to eight ounces of water every 10 to 15 minutes during the workout.

**NOTE:** A sports drink that contains no more than 10 percent carbohydrates may be substituted for water. More than 10 percent will interfere with fluid absorption in the stomach and should not be used.

## Fiber

Even though fiber is not considered a nutrient, it's worth mentioning here. It is indigestible and supplies no calories. Many doctors believe that eating food naturally high in fiber reduces the transit time of fecal contents, thereby reducing bile levels in the intestinal tract, reducing the risk of colon cancer, and reducing the amount of cholesterol absorbed into the bloodstream. High-fiber foods such as whole grains, fruits, and vegetables are also naturally low in fat. The average American consumes only about 10 to 12 grams of fiber daily. If you adhere to the four-food-group system and eat four servings of breads and cereal as well as four servings of fruits and vegetables, you would get about 16 grams of fiber daily.

## SECTION 4.3    THE MEAL PLAN

This chapter presents many charts and tables outlining what you should and shouldn't eat. You've been given the information on what food is good for your body, food that will promote fat loss and muscle gains. You've got to turn that into a system that will work in your life right now.

I cringe when I hear a client say, "I'm on a diet." To me, that implies a temporary change in eating habits that accomplishes just that—a temporary change (at best) in the body and, more than likely, a loss of lean muscle tissue. We're looking for a positive and permanent change.

This book is about looking at exercise, food, and *life* differently. You've come this far in making the decision to improve your body and your life. Embarking on an exercise program is truly the best thing you'll ever do for yourself. However, in order for exercise to be effective, you have to back up your workouts with a solid nutritional program that's doable on a daily basis. Otherwise, it's worthless.

I'm reminded of a firefighter I used to train whose love for training was surpassed only by his love for eating. Dominic was in the gym every day, doing whatever I'd suggest and with a real passion. He continued to make increases in strength, but his appearance never changed in the three months we'd been working together. We finally took a close look at his eating habits and realized that *no* level of training could ever offset his 5,000-calorie-a-day diet, which included everything from cheeseburgers and french fries to boxes of chocolate after dinner. Obviously, an adjustment had to be made, and once it was, the fat melted off Dom's body and revealed all that muscle he'd been hiding underneath.

Let's start at the beginning. Most Americans underestimate their caloric intake. What are you eating now? Begin your new outlook on food by taking a close look at what you now eat. For one full week, keep a *food diary* of everything you put into your mouth, estimating serving sizes and calories. Include everything you eat *and* drink because liquids (except for water) tend to be high in calories. Charting your food intake takes the guesswork out of creating a program that's at least an improvement over your present eating habits. Feel free to copy and use the blank meal plan chart presented in Appendix C. Remember that the goal is to improve on what you're now eating, not to live up to anyone else's standard or to achieve perfection.

We all have different daily caloric requirements based on activity levels and natural metabolic rates.

The number of calories consumed daily must be adjusted to fit individual needs. It's not something you can just look up on some chart. Fit, active people usually need more food than sedentary, out-of-shape people. For example, a very athletic woman might be able to maintain her body weight at 3,000 calories a day. Another woman who is quite sedentary might gain body fat at 1,500 calories a day. You have to determine what you're consuming now and work from there. If you consume foods low in fat and refined sugars and continue to exercise, you'll be sure to lose body fat. Keep in mind that exercise will increase your daily caloric expenditure and metabolic rate.

Normally, just taking a close look at your daily diet will result in improving your eating habits. The next step is to plan meals in advance using the four-food-group system as a guide to your daily intake. Many small meals (up to six) are preferable to two or three large meals, as your body is able to assimilate only a certain amount of nutrients at a time and will turn the rest to fat. When planning, be sure to select foods from all four food groups each day.

Make any changes in your daily diet regimen gradually. Dramatically cutting your caloric intake would undoubtedly slow down your metabolism and force your body to conserve energy in the form of *fat*. Take things one step at a time and one day at a time, giving your body a chance to adapt to your new program.

Another great way to cut unwanted calories is to eliminate most garnishes in the nonfood group. These are a hidden source of unwanted fat and sugar that you sometimes don't even realize you're consuming. Learn to use butter, salad dressings, mayonnaise and the like sparingly, if at all. Substitute with flavorful alternatives or simply use a small amount of the real thing. I recall a saying my mother often repeated to me at the dinner table: *"Everything in moderation."* Those are words of great wisdom, especially when applied to what you eat.

## Sample Meal Plans

This section presents some sample meal plans to help you get started. These three daily sample meal plans are based on the four-food-group system. The first sample plan is for the more sedentary person with a lower daily caloric requirement. The last plan is for someone who works out, leads a more active life, and needs more calories every day. The middle plan suits the average individual who's somewhere in between. Remember, these are only guidelines, not hard and fast rules. You're encouraged to adapt these charts to fit your own dietary regimen and to use them as a way to track and improve on what you now eat. See Appendix C for a blank meal plan chart.

Be sure to include any additional calories you consume from the following sources:

▶ All liquids excluding water and diet beverages
▶ Calories added to foods in the form of oils, butter, gravies, dressings, and the like

**NOTE:**
Handy booklets with calorie-counting charts listing the protein, carbohydrate, and fat content of almost every food can be purchased at most book stores and can also be found at your local supermarket checkout counter.

## FIGURE 4.2    FOUR-FOOD-GROUP SAMPLE MEAL PLAN—LOW CALORIE.

| Meal/Time | Foods | Calories | Protein (g) | Carbs (g) | Fat (g) | Food Group |
|---|---|---|---|---|---|---|
| **BREAKFAST** | | | | | | |
| 7:00 AM | ¾ CUP OATMEAL | 109 | 6.5 | 19 | 2 | GRAIN |
| | 1 CUP SKIM MILK | 86 | 8.4 | 11.9 | 0.4 | MILK |
| | 1 CUP COTTAGE CHS | 160 | 28 | 3.1 | 2.5 | MILK |
| **SNACK** | | | | | | |
| 10:00 AM | 1 PC. WHOLE FRUIT | 80 | 0.5 | 22 | 0.2 | VEG |
| **LUNCH** | | | | | | |
| 1:00 PM | 3½ OZ TURKEY BRST | 140 | 30 | 0 | 2.1 | MEAT |
| | 1 ENGLISH MUFFIN | 154 | 5.1 | 30 | 2.6 | GRAIN |
| **SNACK** | | | | | | |
| 4:00 PM | ¾ CUP VEG JUICE | 74 | 2 | 17.1 | 0.6 | VEG |
| **DINNER** | | | | | | |
| 6:00 PM | 3 OZ BROILED FISH | 100 | 21 | 0 | 1 | MEAT |
| | ½ CUP BRN RICE | 110 | 2.5 | 25 | 1 | GRAIN |
| | 1 CUP STM BROCCOLI | 44 | 5 | 8 | 0.6 | VEG |
| | ½ CUP GARD SALAD | 33 | 2.6 | 7 | 2.1 | VEG |
| | LO-CAL DRESSING | 32 | 0 | 1.5 | 3 | NONFOOD |
| **SNACK** | | | | | | |
| 8:00 PM | 1 CUP STRWBRIES | 45 | 1 | 10 | 0.5 | VEG |
| | 1 OZ HARD PRTZL | 125 | 3 | 24 | 1.5 | GRAIN |
| **TOTALS** | | **1292** | **83** | **179** | **21** | |

### Daily Comments

| | | |
|---|---|---|
| Meat group: | 2 | Only nonfood all day was low-fat dressing w/dinner. |
| Milk group: | 2 | |
| Grain group: | 4 | |
| Vegetable group: | 5 | |
| Nonfood group (fat/oil/sugar): | 1 | |

## FIGURE 4.3    FOUR-FOOD-GROUP SAMPLE MEAL PLAN—MEDIUM CALORIE.

| Meal/Time | Foods | Calories | Protein (g) | Carbs (g) | Fat (g) | Food Group |
|-----------|-------|----------|-------------|-----------|---------|------------|
| **BREAKFAST** | | | | | | |
| 6:00 AM | 1 CUP DRY CEREAL | 100 | 2 | 24 | 0 | GRAIN |
| | 1 CUP SKIM MILK | 80 | 8.4 | 12 | 0.5 | MILK |
| | ¼ CUP RAISINS | 109 | 1.2 | 28 | 0.2 | VEG |
| | ¾ CUP FRUIT JUICE | 74 | 2 | 17.1 | 0.6 | VEG |
| **SNACK** | | | | | | |
| 9:00 AM | 1 CUP L/F YOGURT | 144 | 12 | 16 | 3.5 | MILK |
| | 1 PC. WHOLE FRUIT | 80 | 0.5 | 22 | 0.2 | VEG |
| **LUNCH** | | | | | | |
| 12 NOON | 3 OZ. TUNA IN WATER | 116 | 22.7 | 0 | 2.1 | MEAT |
| | L/F MAYO | 50 | 0.2 | 0.2 | 6 | NONFOOD |
| | LETT/TOMATO SLCD | 60 | 0.5 | 22 | 0.2 | VEG |
| | WW BREAD 2 SLICES | 135 | 4.2 | 28 | 0.14 | GRAIN - 2 |
| **SNACK** | | | | | | |
| 3:00 PM | PROTEIN BAR (WHEY) | 220 | 30 | 20 | 2 | MILK |
| **DINNER** | | | | | | |
| 6:00 PM | 6 OZ TURKEY GRILLED | 266 | 26 | 0 | 6 | MEAT - 2 |
| | 1 BAKED POTATO | 220 | 5 | 51 | 0.2 | VEG |
| | L/F SOUR CREAM | 30 | 1 | 1 | 3 | NONFOOD |
| | 1 CORN (EAR) | 85 | 3 | 20 | 1 | GRAIN |
| **SNACK** | | | | | | |
| 8:00 PM | GRANOLA BAR | 110 | 2.4 | 16 | 4.2 | GRAIN |
| **TOTALS** | | **1900** | **120** | **277** | **27** | |

### Daily Comments

| | | |
|---|---|---|
| Meat group: | 3 | *Good food day. Really enjoyed each meal.* |
| Milk group: | 3 | |
| Grain group: | 5 | |
| Vegetable group: | 5 | |
| Nonfood group (fat/oil/sugar): | 2 | |

## FIGURE 4.4   FOUR-FOOD-GROUP SAMPLE MEAL PLAN—HIGH CALORIE.

| Meal/Time | Foods | Calories | Protein (g) | Carbs (g) | Fat (g) | Food Group |
|---|---|---|---|---|---|---|
| **BREAKFAST** | | | | | | |
| 8:00 AM | 3 WHOLE EGGS | 225 | 19 | 2 | 15 | MEAT |
| | WW BREAD 2 SLICES | 135 | 4.2 | 28 | 0.14 | GRAIN - 2 |
| **SNACK** | | | | | | |
| 11:00 AM | PRTN SHAKE (WHEY) | 300 | 42 | 25 | 2 | MILK - 2 |
| | 1 WHOLE BANANA | 105 | 1.2 | 26.7 | 0.6 | VEG |
| **LUNCH** | | | | | | |
| 2:00 PM | 3 OZ GRILL BURGER | 275 | 12.5 | 30 | 12 | MEAT |
| | LETT/TOM SLICED | 80 | 0.5 | 22 | 0.2 | VEG |
| | 1 HAMBURGER BUN | 119 | 3 | 19.6 | 3.1 | GRAIN - 2 |
| | 1 CUP SOUP CK/RICE | 127 | 12.3 | 13 | 3.2 | GRAIN |
| **SNACK** | | | | | | |
| 5:00 PM | 1 CUP L/F YOGURT | 144 | 12 | 16 | 3.5 | MILK |
| **DINNER** | | | | | | |
| 7:00 PM | 6 OZ CK BRST GRLD | 284 | 54 | 0 | 6.2 | MEAT - 2 |
| | 1 CUP ASPARAGUS | 44 | 5 | 8 | 0.6 | VEG |
| | 2 CUPS CKD PASTA | 394 | 13.2 | 80 | 2 | GRAIN - 2 |
| | ½ CUP TOM. SAUCE | 37 | 1.6 | 8.8 | 0.2 | VEG |
| | 1 GARDEN SALAD | 33 | 2.6 | 7 | 2.1 | VEG |
| | LO-CAL DRESSING | 32 | 0 | 1.5 | 3 | NONFOOD |
| **SNACK** | | | | | | |
| 8:00 PM | 1 CUP FRT CKTAIL | 114 | 1.1 | 29.4 | 0 | VEG |
| REWARD | 2 TBLSPS WHP CRM | 19 | 0.2 | 0.9 | 1.5 | NONFOOD |
| **TOTALS** | | **2467** | **184.4** | **317.9** | **55** | |

### Daily Comments

| | | |
|---|---|---|
| Meat group: | 4 | Needed the extra food due to increased workouts. |
| Milk group: | 3 | |
| Grain group: | 7 | |
| Vegetable group: | 6 | |
| Nonfood group (fat/oil/sugar): | 2 | |

# RED HOOK

When we made the right turn onto that crowded city street, I was hit with a scene I'll never forget. Smoke was pouring from every window of a three-story attached frame building, and so were the children. It was a midsummer morning, and the tight block was lined with people waving us in. A frantic effort was already being made by the firefighters on the scene to reach the trapped kids in any way possible. It was simply a matter of being outnumbered. There were just too many children at too many windows for the firefighters to get to all of them at once.

Arriving at the front of the building, my unit was ordered by the chief running the rescue effort to assist in the removal of some of the children with a portable ladder. At the same time, the bigger but unfortunately slower aerial ladder truck was being prepared to swing into action. The fire inside the building continued to burn out of control. Dense black smoke chased the children to the edge of their windowsills as they choked on their own cries for help.

It became a race to see whether the kids could hold on for the seconds it would take the firemen to get the ladders in position. Because of their heroic and unyielding efforts, the firefighters won the race. On that hot summer morning a half dozen little children were safely plucked from that wood-frame tinderbox with no more than a scratch.

Due to their overall preparedness and ability to handle a crisis, the firefighters of New York City continue to rise to the occasion and go above and beyond the call of duty. This was a clear-cut example of what mental and physical preparation, in the form of *training*, can allow someone to accomplish.

## Review

▷ Avoid unhealthy, nutrient-deficient fad diets that might rob you of lean muscle mass.

▷ Use body-fat assessment as a way to evaluate the progress of your nutrition and exercise program.

▷ Use the four-food-group system as a guide to your daily food intake.

| | | |
|---|---|---|
| Group 1 | Meat | Two or three daily servings |
| Group 2 | Milk | Two or three daily servings |
| Group 3 | Grains | At least four daily servings |
| Group 4 | Vegetables | At least four daily servings |
| Nonfood group | Fats, oils, sweets | Use sparingly |

▷ Ensure that you're getting an adequate supply of protein, carbohydrates, vitamins, minerals, and fiber. If you adhere to the four-food-group system this will happen automatically.

▷ Drink three or four quarts of water daily. Ensure that you're well hydrated before, during, and after exercise.

▷ Take a close look at what you presently eat and make every effort to improve upon that.

▷ Using one of the sample meal plan charts as a guide, record what you eat every day using a blank chart (see Appendix C).

▷ Adjust your caloric intake to fit your metabolism and activity levels.

▷ If at all possible, plan your meals in advance.

▷ This has been said thousands of times by thousands of people, but don't smoke, and drink alcohol only in moderation (a lot of hidden calories there).

▷ Get the advice of your physician before making any major changes in your present diet.

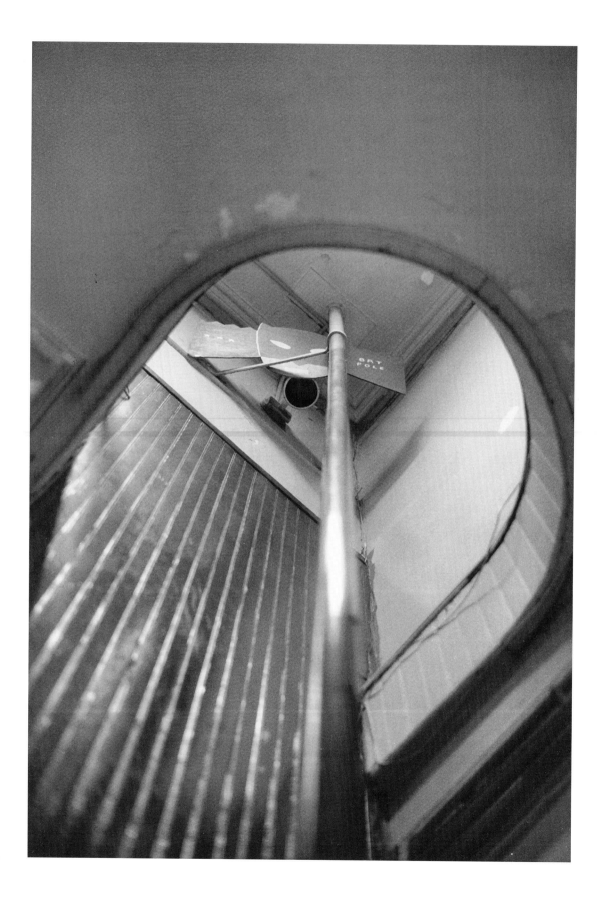

# Exercises and Routines

## SECTION 5.1   STRENGTH-TRAINING EXERCISES

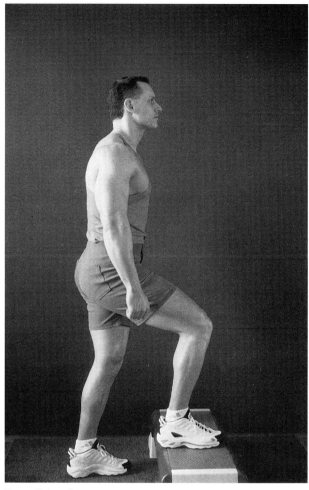

Figure 5.1*a*   Step-up.

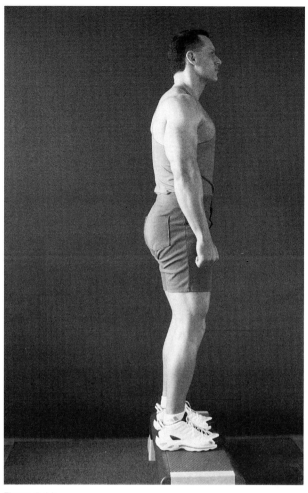

Figure 5.1*b*

## EXERCISE 1   STEP-UP

*Legs and buttocks (quads, hamstrings, and gluteus)*

1. Place your right foot flat on the step and your left foot flat on the floor (Figure 5.1*a*).
2. *Exhale* and push off as little as possible with the left foot as you bring both feet up to step level (you'll now have two feet on the step; see Figure 5.1*b*).
3. *Inhale* and lower your left foot to the floor and repeat.

Repeat with the legs reversed.

*Repetitions:* 10 to 20 on each side.

**TRAINER'S NOTES:**
You can hold dumbbells in your hands for added intensity and balance. I like this one as a home exercise, because it requires only moderate weight to get results as compared to various other leg exercises.

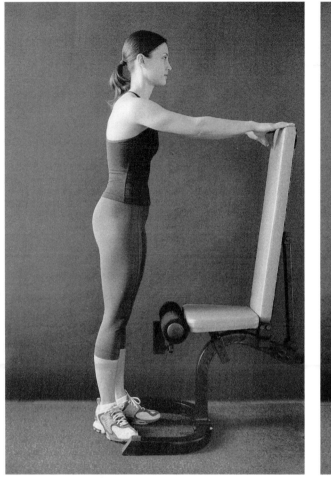

Figure 5.2*a*  Standing Kickback.

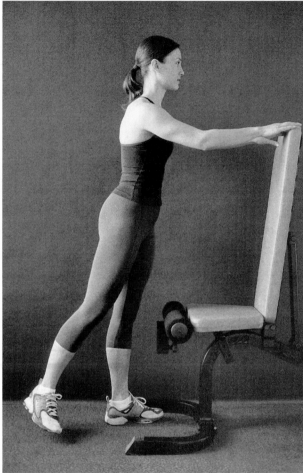

Figure 5.2*b*

## EXERCISE 2  STANDING KICKBACK
*Buttocks (gluteus)*

1. Stand holding the back of a chair or bench for balance. With your feet together, rotate your right foot to the right with all the rotation coming from your hip joint (Figure 5.2*a*).
2. *Exhale* and in a very slow and controlled motion with the right foot rotated out, without bending your knee, lift the right leg (with all motion at the hip joint) behind you (Figure 5.2*b*). The actual movement will be only a slight lift.

3. *Inhale* and slowly lower leg to starting position.

*Repetitions:*  10 to 15

### TRAINER'S NOTES:
Repeat on the other leg. Ankle weights can be added to increase resistance. This movement is aimed primarily at the gluteus muscle (buttocks). In order to isolate the target muscle totally, make sure all the motion is coming from the hip joint with all movements being very slow and controlled. A brief hold at the top of the movement will increase the intensity.

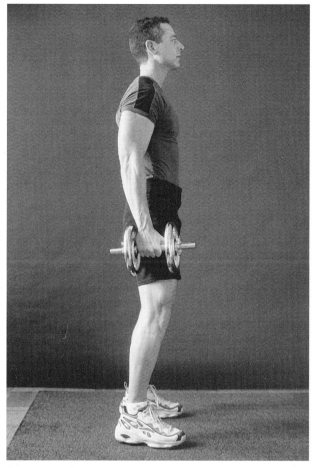

Figure 5.3*a* Squat with Dumbbells.

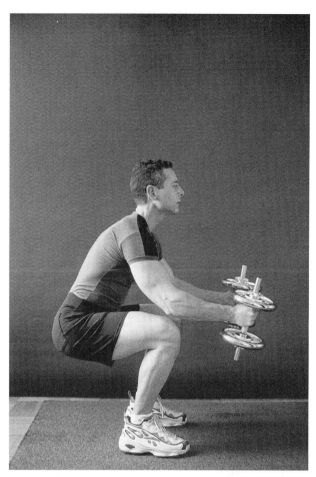

Figure 5.3*b*

## EXERCISE 3   SQUAT WITH DUMBBELLS
*Legs and buttocks (quadriceps, hamstrings, and gluteus)*

1. Stand with your feet shoulder width apart or slightly wider, holding selected dumbbells at your sides. Hold your head straight; maintain the natural arch in your back (Figure 5.3*a*).
2. *Inhale*, swinging the weights slightly forward for balance while bending at the knees and hips to a sitting position, thighs parallel to the floor (or as low as you can safely go while maintaining balance). Your buttocks do not drop below the level of your knees, and your knees do not extend beyond the toes (Figure 5.3*b*).

3. *Exhale*, slowly rising to a standing position with knees and hips straight, allowing the dumbbells to drop back to your sides.

*Repetitions:* 8 to 15

### TRAINER'S NOTES:
Squats are a great movement for the *entire lower body*, bringing all the muscles of legs and buttocks into play as well as the stabilizer muscles of the abdomen and lower back. To increase the intensity without adding weight, squat down to a count of 8 and up to count of 4 (versus the normal 4 down and 2 up).

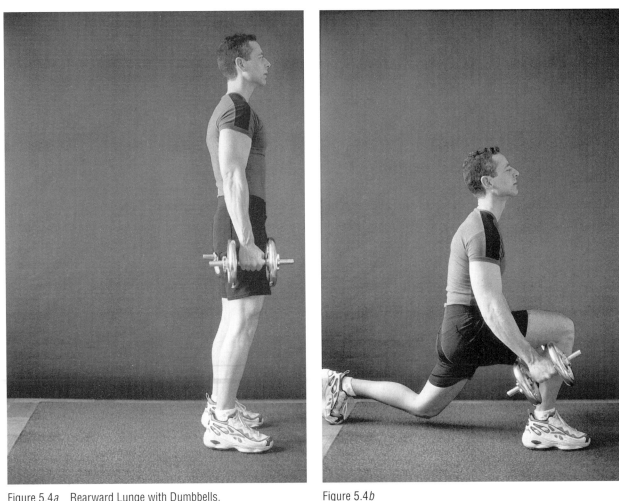

Figure 5.4*a*   Rearward Lunge with Dumbbells.          Figure 5.4*b*

## EXERCISE 4   REARWARD LUNGE WITH DUMBBELLS

*Legs and buttocks (quads, hamstrings, and gluteus)*

1. Stand with feet shoulder width apart, holding one dumbbell in each hand (Figure 5.4*a*).
2. *Inhale* and take a large step backward with the *left foot* to a point where your *left knee* is a few inches above the floor, and your right knee does not extend beyond the toes of your right foot. Hands remain at your sides; gaze forward (Figure 5.4*b*).
3. *Exhale* and step forward with the left leg, returning to the starting position. Finish all reps with the left leg before repeating with the right.

*Repetitions:*  8 to 15

### TRAINER'S NOTES:

This movement not only builds muscle but also works on balance, which is an integral part of functional fitness. Using heavier dumbbells will increase the intensity, while alternating legs from rep to rep instead of set to set will decrease it.

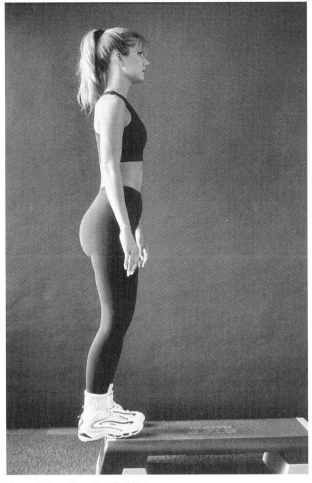

Figure 5.5*a*    Standing Calf Raise.

Figure 5.5*b*

## EXERCISE 5    STANDING CALF RAISE
*Calves*

1. Stand on the end of your step or calf machine with the front half of both feet, heels hanging over the edge (Figure 5.5*a*).
2. *Exhale*, bending only at the ankle joint, and rise up on your toes, pushing hard at the top of the movement (Figure 5.5*b*).
3. *Inhale* and slowly lower your heels, feeling the stretch in your calves.

*Repetitions:* 15 to 20

**TRAINER'S NOTES:**
Calves need to be worked in a higher repetition range than most other muscles (at least 15 reps). To increase intensity levels without increasing weight, use slow and controlled movements, getting a good stretch at the bottom of the movement and pushing hard at the top. This movement can also be performed with one leg at a time to increase the intensity.

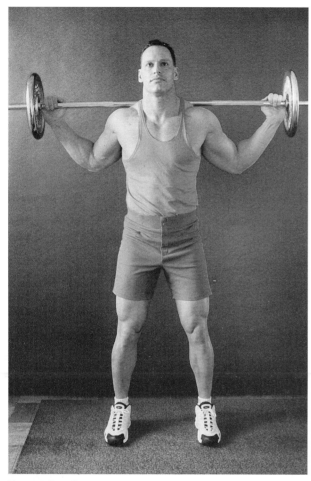

Figure 5.6*a*   Squat with Barbell.

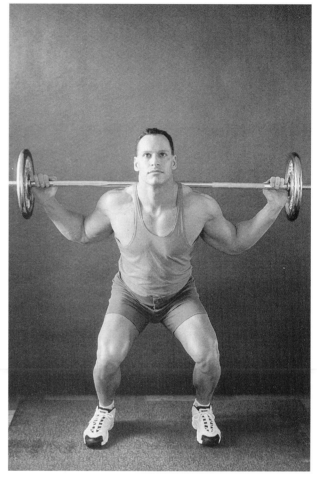

Figure 5.6*b*

## EXERCISE 6   SQUAT WITH BARBELL

*Thighs and buttocks (quadriceps, hamstrings, and gluteus)*

1. Stand with your feet shoulder width apart (or slightly wider), with the bar resting across your shoulders. Hold your head straight; maintain the natural arch in your back (Figure 5.6*a*).
2. *Inhale,* bending at the knees and hips to a sitting position, thighs parallel to the floor (or as low as you can safely go while maintaining balance). Your buttocks do not drop below the level of your knees, and your knees do not extend beyond the toes (Figure 5.6*b*).
3. *Exhale,* slowly rising to a standing position with knees and hips aligned.

*Repetitions:* 8 to 15

### TRAINER'S NOTES:

When using heavier weight, pad the bar as it rests across your shoulders. Ensure that your knees do not extend beyond the toes when at the bottom of the movement.

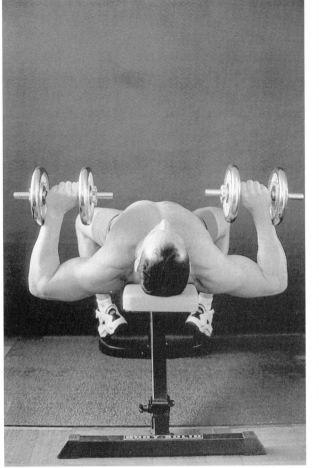

Figure 5.7*a* Bench Press with Dumbbells.

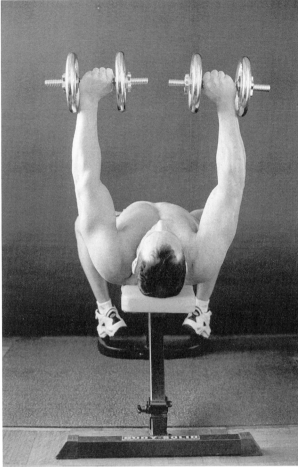

Figure 5.7*b*

## EXERCISE 7 BENCH PRESS WITH DUMBBELLS
*Chest, shoulders, and arms (pectorals, deltoids, and triceps)*

1. Lie supine (flat on your back) on your bench, holding dumbbells at your shoulders, elbows bent, feet planted firmly on the floor. Your shoulders should remain pressed against the bench; maintain a slight arch in your lower back throughout the movement (Figure 5.7*a*).
2. *Exhale* and press both dumbbells straight up toward the ceiling (Figure 5.7*b*).
3. *Inhale* and slowly lower weights to the starting position.

*Repetitions:* 8 to 15

### TRAINER'S NOTES:
To increase intensity, perform the lift very slowly, to a count of 4 on the exhalation phase and 8 on the inhalation phase.

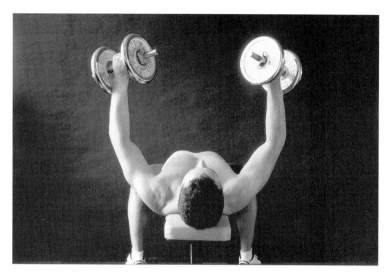

Figure 5.8*a*

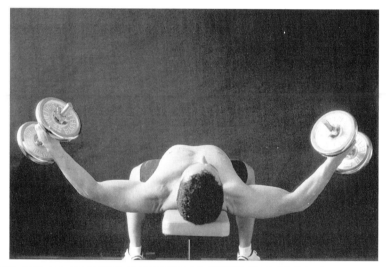

Figure 5.8*b*   Fly with Dumbbells.

## EXERCISE 8   FLY WITH DUMBBELLS
*Chest and shoulders (pectorals and deltoids)*

1. Lie supine on your bench, holding dumbbells above your chest, with elbows slightly bent. Your shoulders should remain pressed against the bench; maintain a slight arch in your lower back throughout the movement (Figure 5.8*a*).
2. *Inhale* as you slowly lower dumbbells in an arch (maintaining the slight bend in the elbow joint) to chest level (Figure 5.8*b*).
3. *Exhale* as you bring the dumbbells together above your chest, still maintaining the slight bend in your elbow.

*Repetitions:* 8 to 15

### TRAINER'S NOTES:
This motion should mimic trying to wrap your arms around a large tree. The same movement can be done on an incline bench.

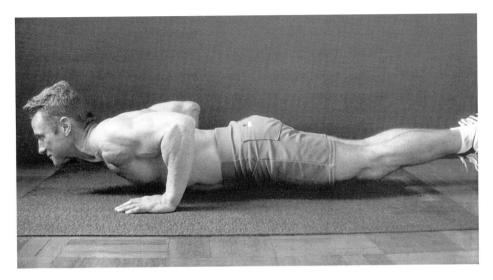

Figure 5.9*a*

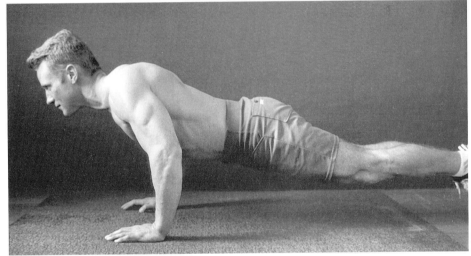

Figure 5.9*b*  Push-up.

## EXERCISE 9  PUSH-UP

*Chest, shoulders, arms, and back (pectorals, deltoids, triceps, and latissimus dorsi)*

1. Lie prone (face down) on the floor or mat; hands on the floor, palms down, slightly wider than shoulder width apart; toes curled under on the floor. Your back and legs are straight (Figure 5.9*a*).
2. *Exhale* as you slowly push your body away from the floor (Figure 5.9*b*).
3. *Inhale*, lowering yourself back down to the point where your chest barely touches or comes to within a few inches of the floor.

*Repetitions:*  Repeat to muscle fatigue.

### TRAINER'S NOTES:

A great exercise that requires no equipment and works virtually your entire upper body. Avoid the tendency to bounce up at the bottom of the motion; use slow and controlled movements throughout.

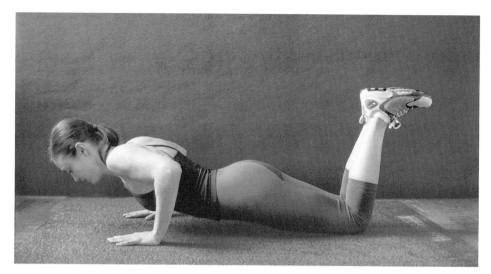

Figure 5.10*a*

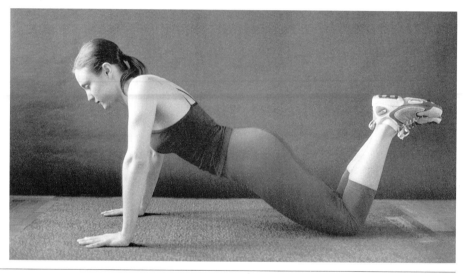

Figure 5.10*b*   Modified Push-up.

## EXERCISE 10   MODIFIED PUSH-UP

*Chest, shoulders, arms, and back (pectorals, deltoids, triceps, and latissimus dorsi)*

Everything remains the same as in the regular push-up, except the knees are bent and remain on the floor throughout the movement instead of the feet (Figure 5.10).

*Repetitions:* Repeat to muscle fatigue.

### TRAINER'S NOTES:

The effectiveness of this movement should not be underestimated as it works the entire upper body simultaneously. It can be modified for men or women.

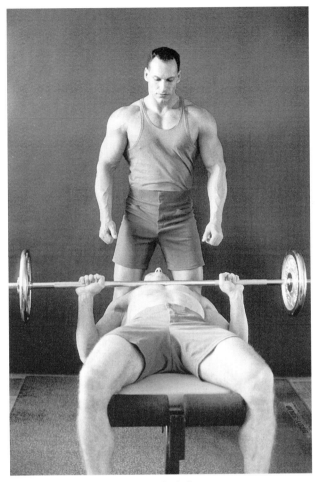

Figure 5.11*a*  Bench Press with Barbell.

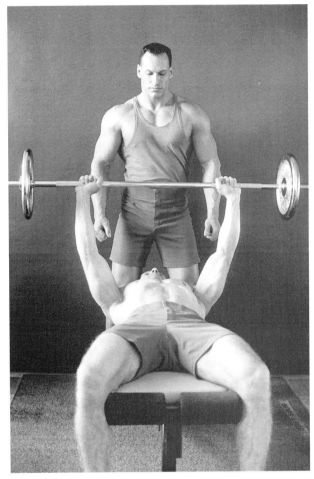

Figure 5.11*b*

# EXERCISE 11  BENCH PRESS WITH BARBELL
*Chest, shoulders, and arms (pectorals, deltoids, and triceps)*

1. Lie supine (flat on your back) on your bench, holding the bar at or slightly wider than shoulder width, feet planted firmly on the floor. Your shoulders should remain pressed against the bench; maintain a slight arch in your lower back throughout the movement (Figure 5.11*a*).
2. *Exhale* and slowly lift the bar straight up toward the ceiling (Figure 5.11*b*).
3. *Inhale* and slowly lower the bar to the middle of your chest (nipple line).

*Repetitions:* 8 to 15

## TRAINER'S NOTES:
To increase intensity perform the lift very slowly, to a count of 4 on the exhalation phase and 8 on the inhalation phase. The "line" of the lift should be from across the middle of your chest at the bottom to a point above your mouth at the top. For safety's sake, I recommend training with a partner any time you do barbell bench presses.

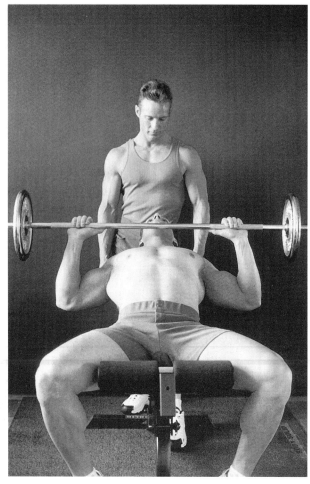

Figure 5.12*a*    Incline Press with Barbell.

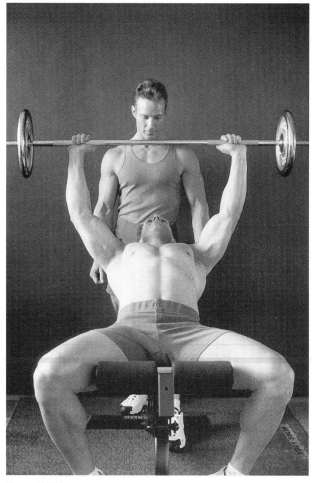

Figure 5.12*b*

## EXERCISE 12    INCLINE PRESS WITH BARBELL
*Chest, shoulders, and arms (pectorals, deltoids, and triceps)*

1. Adjust your bench so the back is at a 45-degree angle to the floor; lie supine (flat on your back), holding the bar at or slightly wider than shoulder width, feet planted firmly on the floor. Your shoulders should remain pressed against the bench; maintain a slight arch in your lower back throughout the movement (Figure 5.12*a*).
2. *Exhale* and slowly push the bar straight up toward the ceiling (Figure 5.12*b*).
3. *Inhale* and slowly lower the bar to the top of your chest.

*Repetitions:* 8 to 15

### TRAINER'S NOTES:
The incline press is a great variation on the bench press and can also be done with dumbbells. Another variation is to use the incline bench to do flies. For safety's sake, I recommend training with a partner when using this exercise.

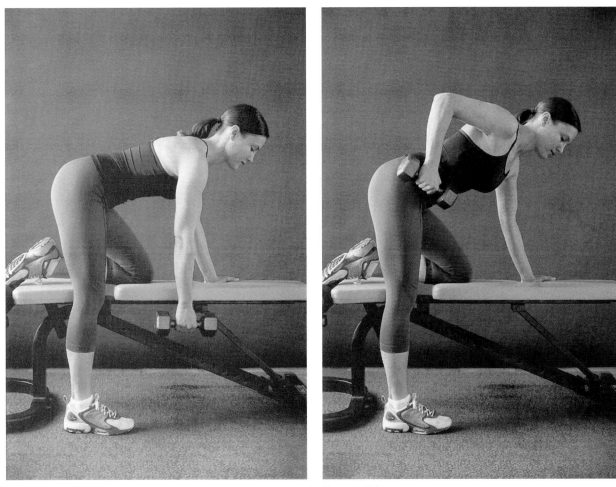

Figure 5.13*a*    Bent Row with Dumbbell.

Figure 5.13*b*

## EXERCISE 13    BENT ROW WITH DUMBBELL
*Back and arms (latissimus dorsi and biceps)*

1. Stand with the right foot on the floor and the left knee on the bench or step as you bend at the waist, holding a dumbbell in the right hand near the floor directly under the right shoulder. Place the left hand on the bench for support (Figure 5.13*a*).
2. *Exhale* as you pull the weight up from the floor to your right hip (Figure 5.13*b*).
3. *Inhale* as you slowly lower to the starting position, making sure to feel the pull at the bottom of the movement.

*Repetitions:* 8 to 15 on each side.

### TRAINER'S NOTES:
With this exercise—as with all back movements— it's important to get full range of motion and stretch. Accomplish this by letting your arm extend fully when lowering the dumbbell.

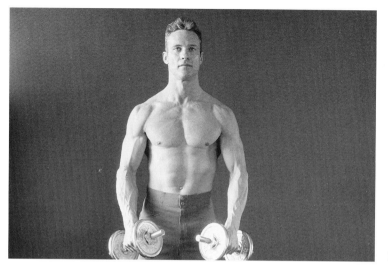

Figure 5.14*a*

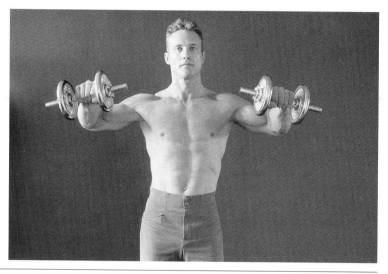

Figure 5.14*b*   Upright Row with Dumbbells.

## EXERCISE 14   UPRIGHT ROW WITH DUMBBELLS

*Upper back, shoulders, and arms (trapezius, deltoids, and biceps)*

1. Stand with feet shoulder width apart, holding dumbbells at waist level, but about six inches out from the body (Figure 5.14*a*).
2. *Exhale* as you keep the weights away from your body and pull up, ensuring that your elbows never rise above shoulder level (Figure 5.14*b*).
3. *Inhale* as you lower dumbbells to the starting position.

*Repetitions:* 8 to 15

### TRAINER'S NOTES:

Be sure to keep the dumbbells at least six inches out from body, reducing any chance of shoulder strain. This movement mimics pulling the starter cord on a lawn mower, only with both arms at once.

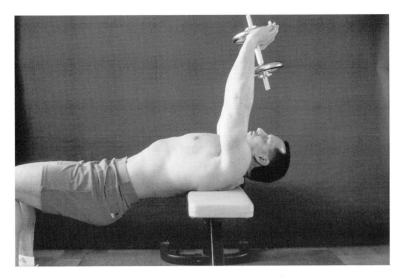

Figure 5.15*a*

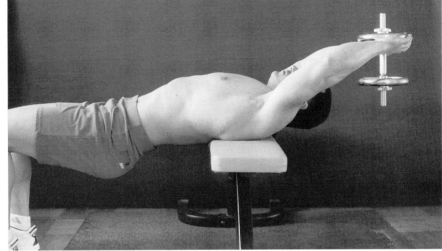

Figure 5.15*b*    Pullover with Dumbbell.

## EXERCISE 15    PULLOVER WITH DUMBBELL

*Back, shoulders, and chest (latissimus dorsi, deltoids, and pectorals)*

1. Lie *across* your bench with both hands above your chest and wrapped around the neck of one dumbbell. Knees are bent, with the feet firmly on the floor; lower back is arched (Figure 5.15*a*).
2. With both elbow joints almost locked, bend only at the shoulder joint while you *inhale* and lower the dumbbell beyond your head and toward the floor (Figure 5.15*b*).
3. *Exhale* as you slowly raise the weight to the starting position.

*Repetitions:* 8 to 15

### TRAINER'S NOTES:

This is a great strength exercise, but also provides a powerful stretch for the shoulder and chest muscles.

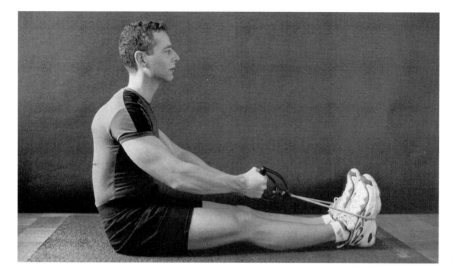

Figure 5.16*a*

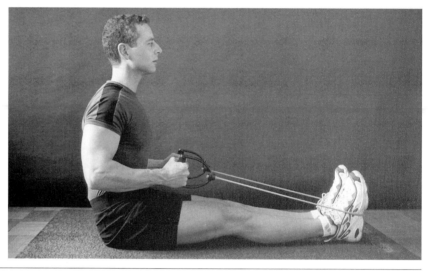

Figure 5.16*b*   Cable Row with
Resistance Tubing.

## EXERCISE 16   CABLE ROW WITH RESISTANCE TUBING

*Back and arms (latissimus dorsi, rhomboids, and biceps)*

1. Sit on the floor with legs straight out in front of you, upper body upright, and the resistance tubing wrapped around the bottom of your feet (Figure 5.16*a*).
3. Grab onto the ends of the tubing with both hands, *exhale,* and pull into your abdomen (Figure 5.16*b*).
3. *Inhale* as you slowly return to the starting position.

*Repetitions:* 8 to 15

**TRAINER'S NOTES:**
Training the back on home equipment can present a unique challenge due to the *pulling* requirements involved in getting a good back workout (versus *pushing* or pressing a weight away from yourself, as in a bench press). Resistance tubing, which comes in various lengths and resistances, satisfies the need perfectly. The resistance tubing can also be used for other movements as well, limited only by your imagination.

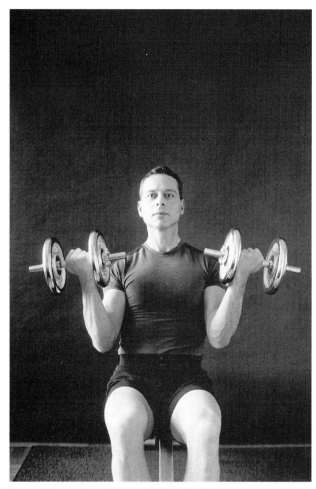

Figure 5.17*a*  Seated Press with Dumbbells.

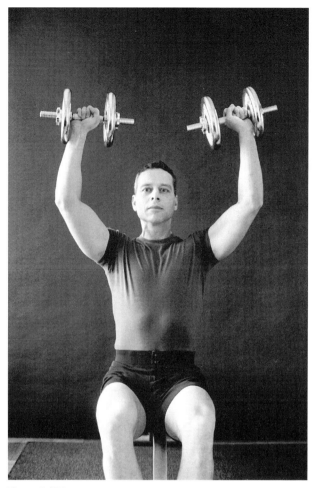

Figure 5.17*b*

## EXERCISE 17  SEATED PRESS WITH DUMBBELLS

*Shoulders and arms (deltoids and triceps)*

1. Sit on the end of your step or bench, holding dumbbells at shoulder level, palms facing toward your body, back straight (Figure 5.17*a*).
2. *Exhale* as you extend your arms overhead, and rotate the dumbbells until the palms face away from your body (Figure 5.17*b*).
3. *Inhale* and slowly lower weights to the starting position.

*Repetitions:* 8 to 15

**TRAINER'S NOTES:**

The twist should go from palms facing rearward at the start to palms forward at the top of the lift. This places the shoulder joint in a more protected position during the lift. This exercise can also be done standing.

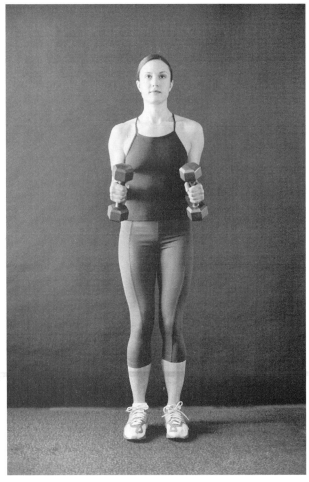

Figure 5.18*a*   Lateral Raise with Dumbbells.

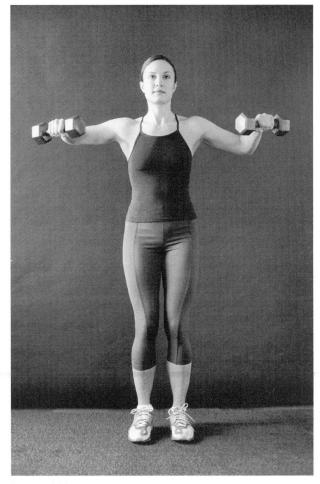

Figure 5.18*b*

## EXERCISE 18   LATERAL RAISE WITH DUMBBELLS

*Shoulders (side and rear deltoids)*

1. Stand with feet shoulder width apart, holding dumbbells at your sides, elbows bent at 90 degrees (as if you were holding two guns at your hips; see Figure 5.18*a*).
2. *Exhale* as you lift your elbows laterally away from your body (Figure 5.18*b*). Make sure the elbows never go above the level of the shoulders.
3. *Inhale* and slowly lower arms to the starting position.

*Repetitions:* 8 to 15

**TRAINER'S NOTES:**
This movement can also be done with elbows straight, but the elbows are kept bent in order to afford protection to the shoulder joint. You'll be able to handle a heavier weight with the elbows bent, and you can increase the intensity simply by using a slightly heavier dumbbell if needed.

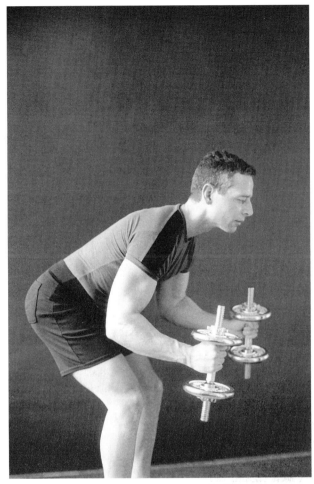

Figure 5.19*a*   Rear Lateral Raise with Dumbbells.

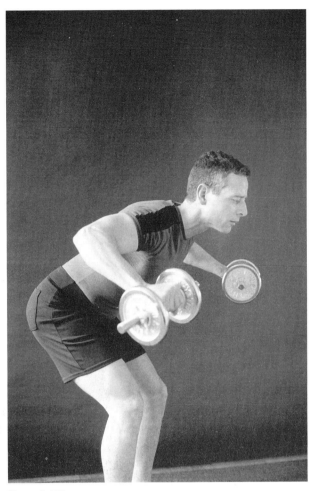

Figure 5.19*b*

# EXERCISE 19   REAR LATERAL RAISE WITH DUMBBELLS

*Shoulders and upper back (rear deltoids and trapezius)*

1. Stand with your feet shoulder width apart, unlock the knees and bend at the waist, holding a dumbbell in each hand, elbows bent at 90 degrees, arms at your sides (Figure 5.19*a*).
2. *Exhale* and bring your upper arms away from your body, maintaining the bend in your elbow (Figure 5.19*b*).

3. *Inhale* and lower arms to the starting position.

*Repetitions:* 8 to 15

### TRAINER'S NOTES:

This is a great movement to isolate the upper-back and rear shoulder muscles. There is a tendency to let the weight drop; be sure to control the weight as it is lowered during the inhalation phase.

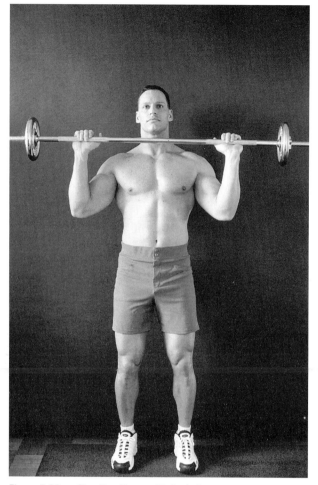

Figure 5.20a   Standing Press with Barbell.

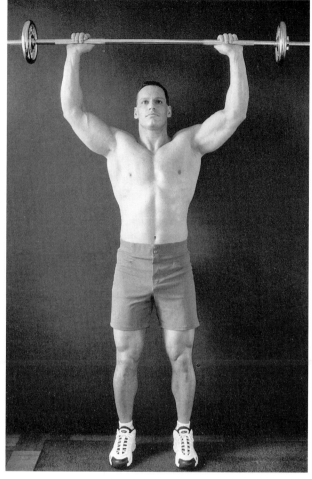

Figure 5.20b

## EXERCISE 20   STANDING PRESS WITH BARBELL

*Shoulders and arms (deltoids and triceps)*

1. Stand in front of the bar, bend at the knees, and grab the bar at shoulder width. Stand straight up as you bring the bar to shoulder level (Figure 5.20a).
2. *Exhale* as you slowly extend your arms, pressing the bar overhead (Figure 5.20b).
3. *Inhale* and slowly lower the bar to the starting position at the front of the body.

*Repetitions:* 8 to 15

### TRAINER'S NOTES:

Be careful not to lean back too far, but maintain the natural arch in your spine when pressing. This exercise can also be done seated on a bench.

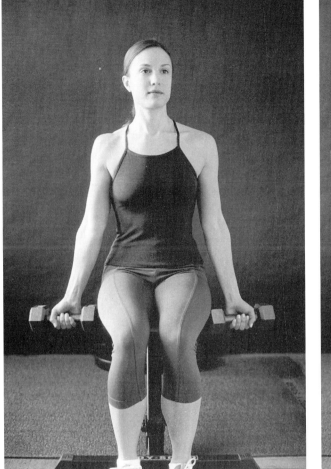

Figure 5.21*a*    Seated Curl with Dumbbells.

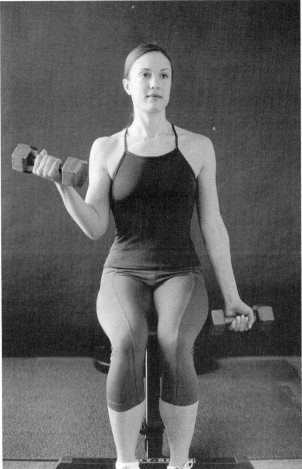

Figure 5.21*b*

## EXERCISE 21    SEATED CURL WITH DUMBBELLS

*Arms (biceps)*

1. Sit on the edge of your bench or step, holding dumbbells at your sides (Figure 5.21*a*).
2. *Exhale* as you slowly curl the right arm up, bending only at the elbow. Make sure you do not swing the weight or use momentum to complete the lift (Figure 5.21*b*).
3. *Inhale* as you curl up the left arm and slowly lower the right. Continue to alternate one arm up, one arm down, breathing with each rep.

*Repetitions:* 8 to 15

**TRAINER'S NOTES:**

This movement may also be done standing or curling both arms together.

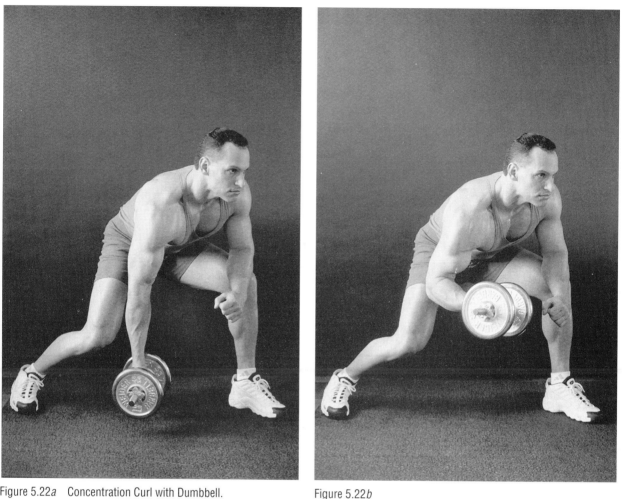

Figure 5.22*a*    Concentration Curl with Dumbbell.

Figure 5.22*b*

## EXERCISE 22    CONCENTRATION CURL WITH DUMBBELL

*Arms (biceps)*

1. Standing, bend at the waist (and slightly at the knees), and let the right arm hang straight down while you hold the selected dumbbell in your right hand. Rest your left elbow on your left knee for support (Figure 5.22*a*).
2. *Exhale* as you slowly curl the right arm up, bending only at the elbow. Make sure you do not swing the weight or use momentum to complete the lift (Figure 5.22*b*).
3. *Inhale* as you slowly lower the dumbbell to the starting position. Repeat with your left arm.

*Repetitions:* 8 to 15

### TRAINER'S NOTES:

Concentration curls are a great way to isolate the biceps.

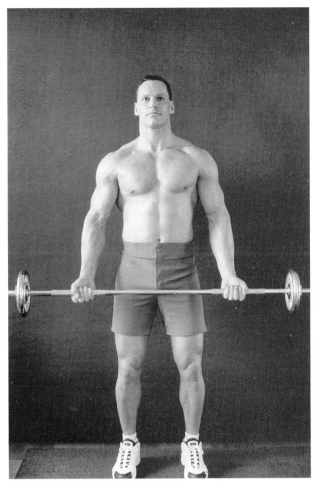

Figure 5.23*a*   Standing Curl with Barbell.

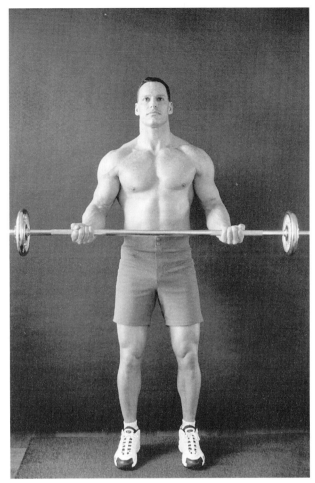

Figure 5.23*b*

## EXERCISE 23   STANDING CURL WITH BARBELL
*Arms (biceps)*

1. Standing, hold the bar in front of you at shoulder width, palms facing forward. Shoulders back; maintain the natural arch in your back; gaze forward (Figure 5.23*a*).
2. *Exhale* as you slowly curl the bar up, bending only at the elbow. The upper arms remain in a fixed position throughout the lift. Make sure you do not swing the bar or use momentum to complete the lift (Figure 5.23*b*).
3. *Inhale* as you slowly lower the bar to the starting position.

*Repetitions:* 8 to 15

### TRAINER'S NOTES:
There is a tendency to jerk and swing the upper body to complete the lift. This will do little to develop the biceps. Use a lighter weight to ensure perfect form and that the biceps are targeted.

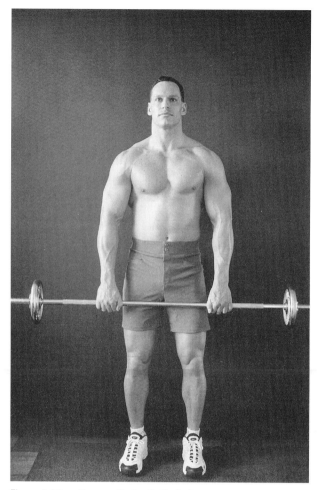

Figure 5.24*a* Reverse Curl with Barbell.

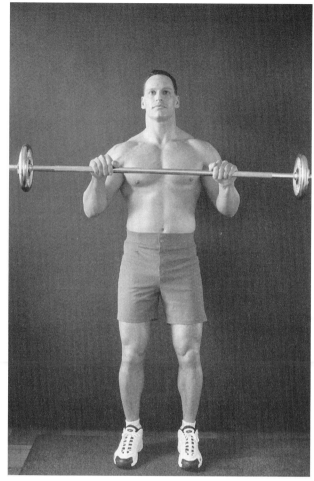

Figure 5.24*b*

## EXERCISE 24   REVERSE CURL WITH BARBELL
*Arms (biceps and forearms)*

1. Standing, hold the bar in front of you, palms facing rearward. Shoulders back; maintain the natural arch in your back; gaze forward (Figure 5.24*a*).
2. *Exhale* as you slowly curl the bar up, bending only at the elbow. The upper arms remain in a fixed position throughout the lift. Make sure you do not swing the bar or use momentum to complete the lift (Figure 5.24*b*).

3. *Inhale* as you slowly lower the bar to the starting position.

*Repetitions:* 8 to 15

### TRAINER'S NOTES:
This is a very similar movement to the barbell curl in Exercise 23 but with the palms facing rearward at the start of the motion, targeting the forearms as well as the biceps.

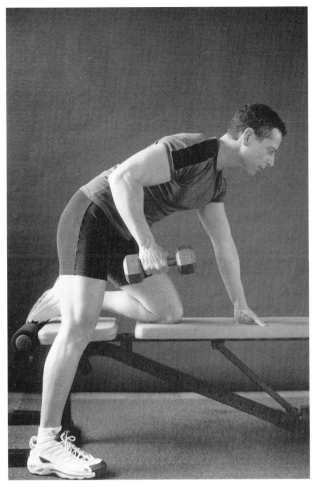

Figure 5.25*a*  Kickback with Dumbbell.

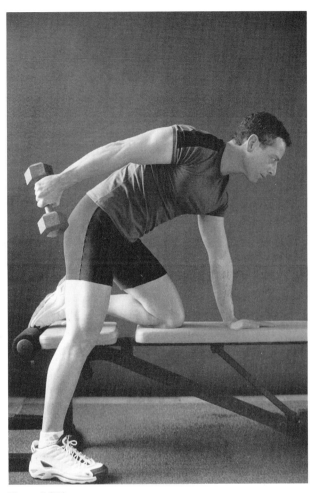

Figure 5.25*b*

## EXERCISE 25  KICKBACK WITH DUMBBELL
*Arms (triceps)*

1. Stand with feet shoulder width apart; bend at the waist with a dumbbell in your right hand, elbow bent. Put your left knee on the bench, and keep your right foot on the floor. Place the left hand on the bench for support (Figure 5.25*a*).
2. With your upper arm parallel to the floor, *exhale* as you straighten the elbow, lifting the weight behind you. Make sure all movement comes from the elbow joint, not the shoulder (Figure 5.25*b*).

3. *Inhale* as you slowly lower the dumbbell to the starting position. Repeat with the left arm.

*Repetitions:* 8 to 15

### TRAINER'S NOTES:
Try not to let the upper arm drop during the lift. Holding the elbow in a steady position will ensure that the triceps gets the full load.

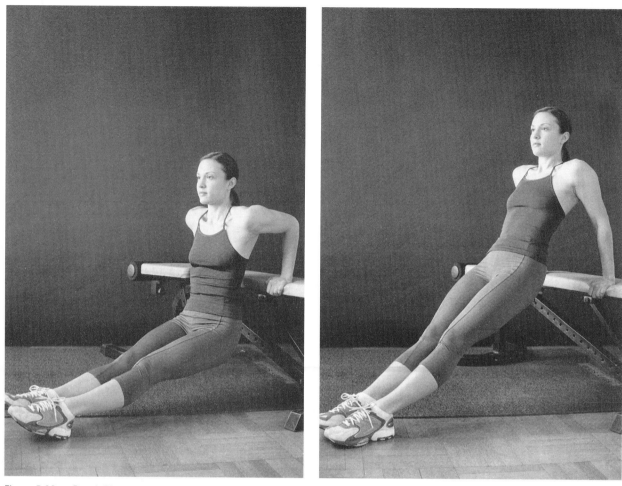

Figure 5.26*a*   Bench Dip.

Figure 5.26*b*

## EXERCISE 26   BENCH DIP
*Arms and shoulders (triceps and deltoids)*

1. Sit off the edge (long side) of your bench or step with your hands on the edge next to your hips, elbows bent. Knees are straight and heels are on the floor. A dumbbell can be placed in your lap for added resistance.
2. Move forward slightly, allowing your buttocks to come off the bench, transferring your body weight to your arms (Figure 5.26*a*).
3. *Exhale* and push down against the bench, lifting yourself up; feet remain on the floor (Figure 5.26*b*).

4. *Inhale* and slowly lower yourself to a point where your buttocks are below the bench; repeat.

*Repetitions:*  8 to 15 with weights; to muscle fatigue without weights

### TRAINER'S NOTES:
This is a great variation on the classic dip but concentrates primarily on the triceps. Intensity can be increased by placing a weight plate or dumbbell in your lap.

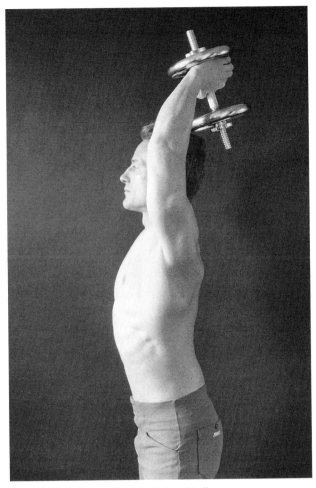

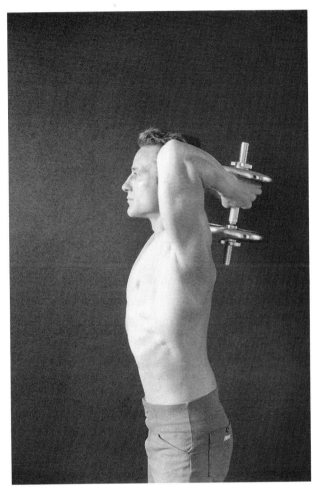

Figure 5.27*a*   Triceps Press with Dumbbell.

Figure 5.27*b*

## EXERCISE 27   TRICEPS PRESS WITH DUMBBELL

*Arms (triceps)*

1. Stand with feet shoulder width apart, holding one dumbbell overhead with both hands; gaze forward (Figure 5.27*a*).
2. *Inhale,* bending only at the elbow joints, and slowly lower the weight behind your head. Make sure all movement comes from the elbow joint and the elbows remain fixed (Figure 5.27*b*).
3. *Exhale* as you straighten your elbows and raise the weight above your head.

*Repetitions:* 8 to 15

**TRAINER'S NOTES:**

Any time you raise a dumbbell above your head, be careful to choose a weight that allows you total control throughout the movement. Be sure to keep the upper arms in a fixed position throughout the lift, thereby increasing the intensity to the target muscle (the tricep).

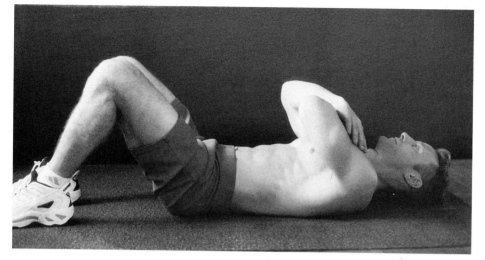

Figure 5.28*a*

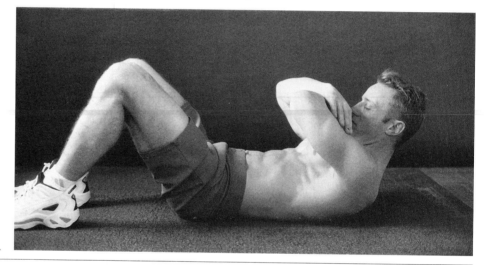

Figure 5.28*b*   Sit-up.

## EXERCISE 28   SIT-UP
*Abdominals and obliques*

1. Lie supine on a mat or padded carpet with your knees *partially* bent, feet flat on the floor, arms folded across your chest (Figure 5.28*a*).
2. *Exhale* as you tighten your buttock muscles and begin to raise your chest off the floor, feeling your abdominal muscles tighten. The movement need only be a few inches (Figure 5.28*b*).
3. *Inhale* as you slowly curl back down without let-ting your head touch the floor, maintaining tension in the abdominal muscles for the entire set.

*Repetitions:* Repeat to muscle fatigue.

### TRAINER'S NOTES:
In order to work the abdominal muscles, only a slight lift of the upper body off the floor is necessary. By keeping your knees slightly bent, the oblique muscles are also brought into play.

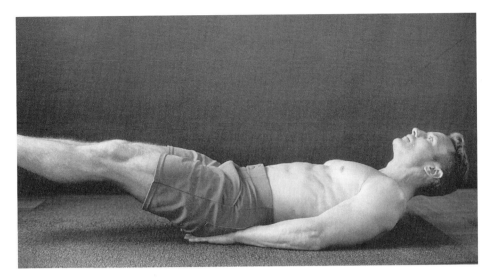

Figure 5.29*a*

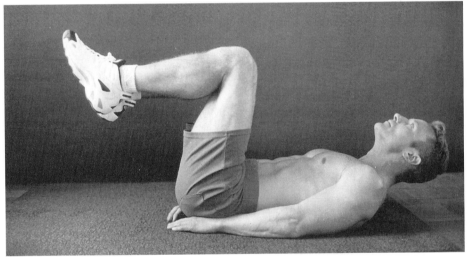

Figure 5.29*b*   Leg Raise.

## EXERCISE 29   LEG RAISE
*Abdominals and hip flexors*

1. Lie supine on a mat or padded carpet, legs straight, both hands under your buttocks to help maintain the proper pelvic tilt, head on the floor (Figure 5.29*a*).
2. *Exhale* as you slowly bring your knees to your chest and your head off the floor (Figure 5.29*b*).
3. *Inhale* as you lower your head and straighten your legs to a point where your feet are a few inches off the floor.

*Repetitions:* Repeat to muscle fatigue.

### TRAINER'S NOTES:
Be sure to keep your hands under your buttocks to ensure the proper pelvic tilt, which will increase the work load on the target muscle as well as protect the lower back from undue strain.

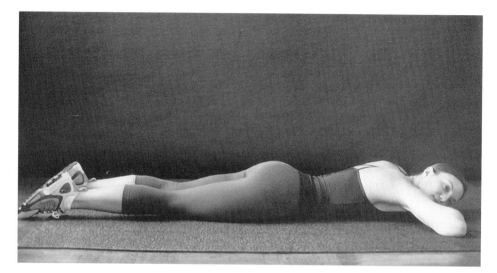

Figure 5.30*a*

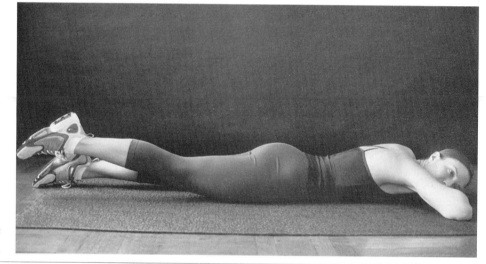

Figure 5.30*b*  Reverse
Leg Raise.

## EXERCISE 30   REVERSE LEG RAISE
*Lower back and buttocks (gluteus)*

1. Lie prone on a mat or padded carpet, head straight. Hands can be used to form a pillow for your face (Figure 5.30*a*).
2. *Inhale* as you slowly raise your right leg without bending the knee, holding briefly at the top of the movement (Figure 5.30*b*).

3. *Exhale* and lower the leg to starting position and repeat. Repeat with the left leg.

*Repetitions:* Repeat to muscle fatigue.

**TRAINER'S NOTES:**
This is actually a yoga movement that's a great muscle builder for the lower back as well.

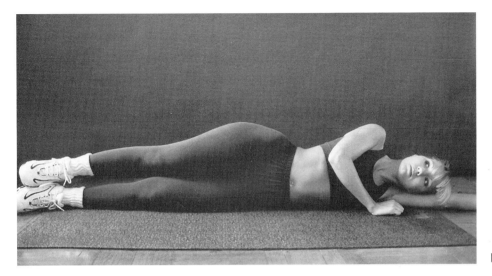

Figure 5.31a

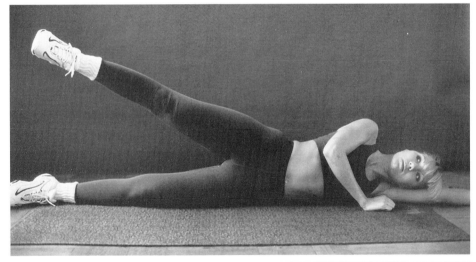

Figure 5.31b   Side Leg Raise.

## EXERCISE 31   SIDE LEG RAISE
*Obliques and hip abductors/adductors*

1. Lie on your left side on a mat or padded carpet, head and legs straight (Figure 5.31a).
2. *Exhale* as you raise your right (top) leg as high as it will comfortably go. All movement comes from the hip joint (Figure 5.31b).

3. *Inhale,* lower top leg to starting position, and repeat. Repeat on the opposite side.

*Repetitions:* Repeat to muscle fatigue.

### TRAINER'S NOTES:
This is a great exercise to develop the oblique muscles that form your waist. And, as an added benefit, it works the inner thigh.

# SECTION 5.2   FLEXIBILITY EXERCISES

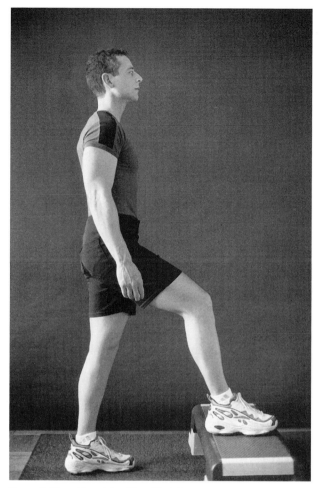

Figure 5.32*a* Hamstring Step Stretch.

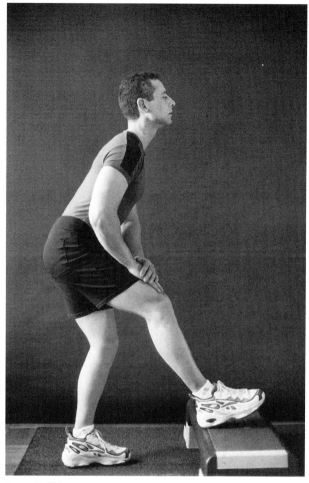

Figure 5.32*b*

## EXERCISE 32    HAMSTRING STEP STRETCH
*Hamstrings*

Stand with your feet shoulder width apart, a foot or two back from your step. Place the heel of the right foot on the step, keeping your left foot planted on the floor (Figure 5.32*a*). *Exhale* and slowly bend the left knee, creating a stretch in the back of the right leg.

You can also bend at the waist and place your hands on your right thigh for support as this will intensify the stretch (Figure 5.32*b*). At the point of *slight discomfort, not pain*, hold the position (this applies to all stretches). *Inhale* and slowly release. Repeat on the opposite leg.

*Hold time:* 15 to 30 seconds

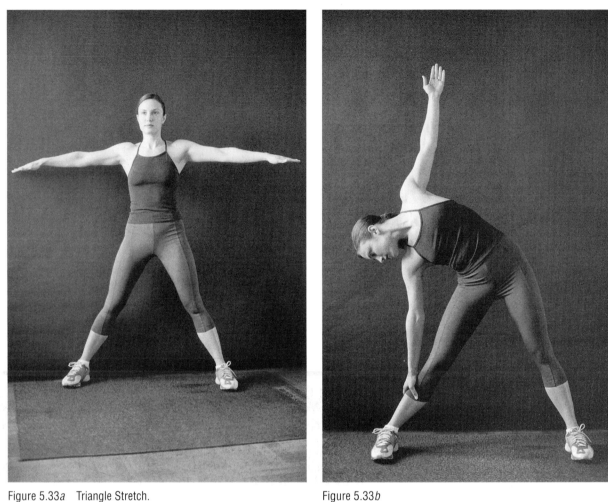

Figure 5.33*a*  Triangle Stretch.

Figure 5.33*b*

## EXERCISE 33   TRIANGLE STRETCH
*Inner thigh*

Stand with your feet wide apart, arms out in a *T* position, and your head straight (Figure 5.33*a*). *Exhale* as you let your upper body drop to the right side, feeling the stretch on the inside of the right leg. Hold the position. For support, your right hand grabs your right leg at the point of natural contact (Figure 5.33*b*). *Inhale* and return to center. Repeat on the left side. This movement may also be performed against a wall to keep the body perfectly aligned.

*Hold time:* 15 to 30 seconds

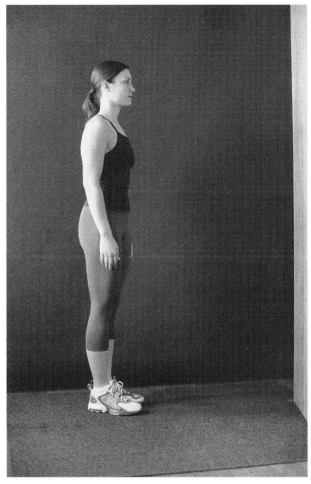

Figure 5.34*a*   Calf Stretch.

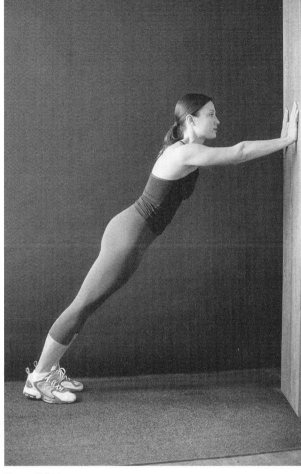

Figure 5.34*b*

## EXERCISE 34   CALF STRETCH
*Calves and Achilles tendons*

Stand with feet together three or four feet out from a wall (Figure 5.34*a*). Place your hands on the wall shoulder width or wider, *exhale* and lean the upper body in toward the wall. Your heels remain planted firmly on the floor as you hold (Figure 5.34*b*). *Inhale* and return to the starting position. One foot can be brought forward to intensify the stretch on the leg that remains planted; repeat on the other side if this is done.

*Hold time:* 15 to 30 seconds

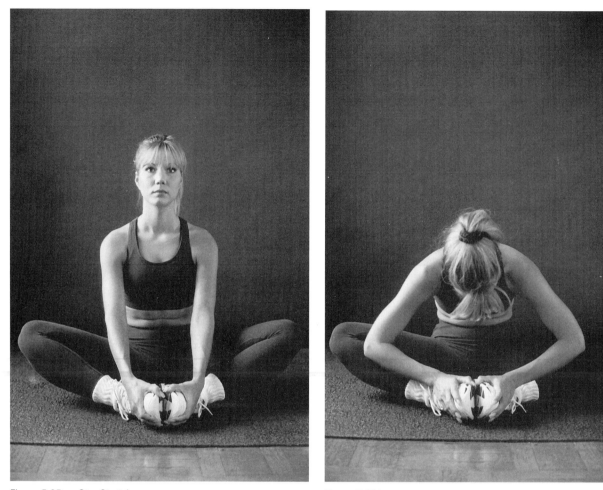

Figure 5.35a  Star Stretch.

Figure 5.35b

## EXERCISE 35   STAR STRETCH
*Back and inner thigh*

Sit on your mat or padded carpet with back straight, knees bent, soles of your feet together. Pull your feet into your body as far as they will comfortably go (Figure 5.35a). Gently rock your legs up and down for a few seconds to loosen your hip joints. *Exhale* as you bend forward, hinging at the waist, pressing the knees down with your elbows. Let your head drop, hold the position, and breathe (Figure 5.35b). *Inhale* and release.

*Hold time:* 15 to 30 seconds

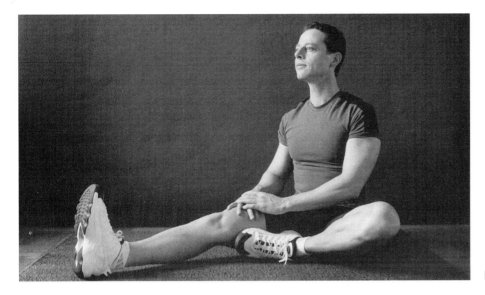

Figure 5.36*a*

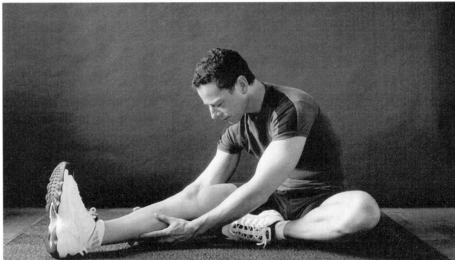

Figure 5.36*b*   Alternate
Leg Stretch.

## EXERCISE 36   ALTERNATE LEG STRETCH
*Hamstrings*

Sit on your mat or padded carpet with the right leg out in front of you (knee straight) and the left leg bent, sole of your left foot resting on your inner thigh (Figure 5.36*a*). *Exhale* and reach up and then over your right leg with both arms as you hinge at the hips. Keep your shoulders relaxed as you grasp the right leg with both hands and hold, feeling the stretch in the back of your right leg (Figure 5.36*b*). *Inhale* and lean back to the starting position. Switch positions with the legs and repeat.

*Hold time:* 15 to 30 seconds

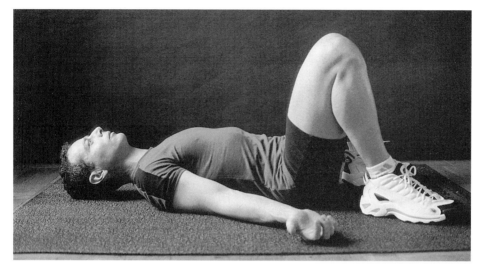

Figure 5.37*a*

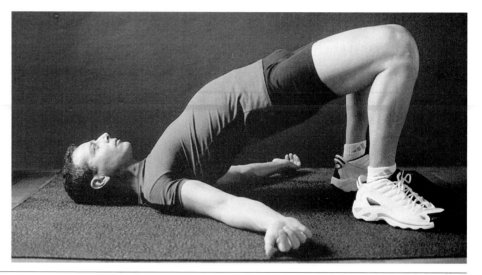

Figure 5.37*b*   The Bridge.

## EXERCISE 37   THE BRIDGE
*Quadriceps, hip flexors, and lower back flex*

Lie on your back on a mat or padded carpet, knees bent, heels near your buttocks, arms at your sides (Figure 5.37*a*). *Inhale* as you slowly raise your pelvis off the floor as high as it will comfortably go. Tighten your buttocks and squeeze your shoulder blades together, hold, and breathe (Figure 5.37*b*). *Exhale* as you lower back down to the floor.

*Hold time:*  10 to 30 seconds

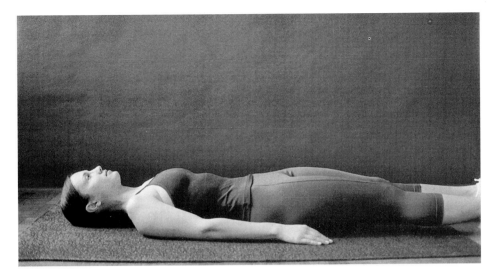

Figure 5.38*a*

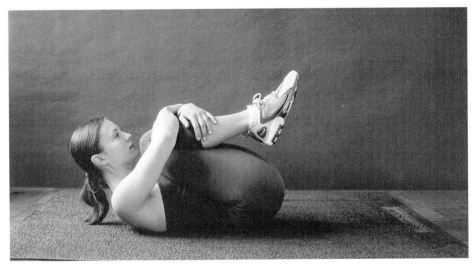

Figure 5.38*b*   Knees-to-Chest
Stretch.

## EXERCISE 38   KNEES-TO-CHEST STRETCH
*Lower back*

Lie supine on your mat or padded carpet, knees straight, arms at your sides (Figure 5.38*a*). *Exhale* as you bring both knees up to your chest. Wrap your arms around both legs and squeeze, making sure your lower back stays on the floor (Figure 5.38*b*). If you experience any knee pain, hold the position by wrapping the arms *under* the knees instead of over the knees. Hold and breathe. *Inhale* as you release.

*Hold time:* 5 to 30 seconds

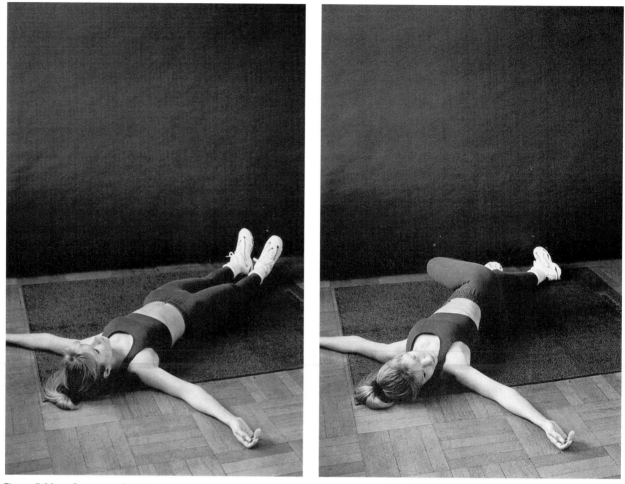

Figure 5.39*a*   Crossover Stretch.

Figure 5.39*b*

## EXERCISE 39   CROSSOVER STRETCH
*Lower back and buttocks*

Lie supine on your mat or padded carpet (Figure 5.39*a*). Place your right foot at your left knee, arms out in a *T*. Place your left hand on your right knee,

*exhale,* and push down while you turn your head to the right (Figure 5.39*b*). Hold briefly. *Inhale* as you release. Repeat with the left leg.

***Hold time:*** 5 to 10 seconds

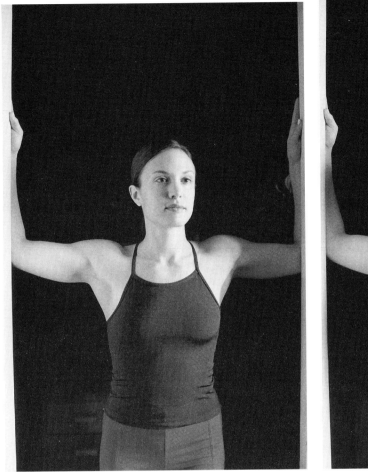

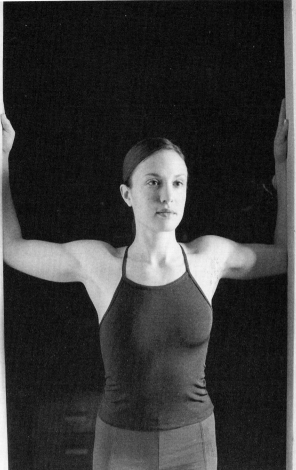

Figure 5.40*a*   Chest Stretch.

Figure 5.40*b*

# EXERCISE 40   CHEST STRETCH
*Chest and shoulders*

Stand in a doorway and place your arms out to your sides, elbows against each side wall (Figure 5.40*a*). *Exhale* and lean your upper body through the doorway as your arms are pushed back and your chest is stretched; hold (Figure 5.40*b*). *Inhale* as you release. This stretch can also be done with one arm at a time. This is an important stretch to maintain a healthy posture of the upper back and eliminate rounded shoulders.

*Hold time:*  15 to 30 seconds

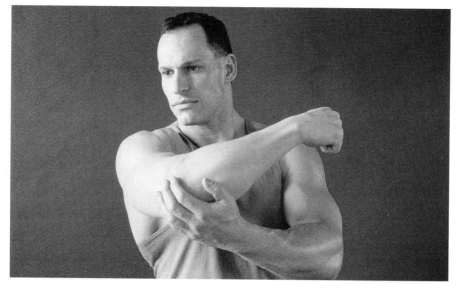

Figure 5.41*a*

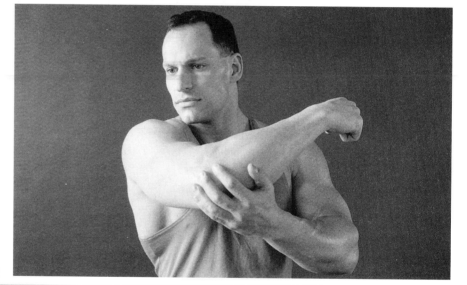

Figure 5.41*b*   Shoulder Crossover.

## EXERCISE 41   SHOULDER CROSSOVER
*Rear shoulders*

Stand or sit and place your right arm across the front of your body at shoulder level (Figure 5.41*a*). Place your left hand on the back of your right elbow, and press your right arm into your body, *exhaling* (Figure 5.41*b*). Hold and breathe. *Inhale* and release. Repeat with your left arm.

*Hold time:* 15 to 30 seconds

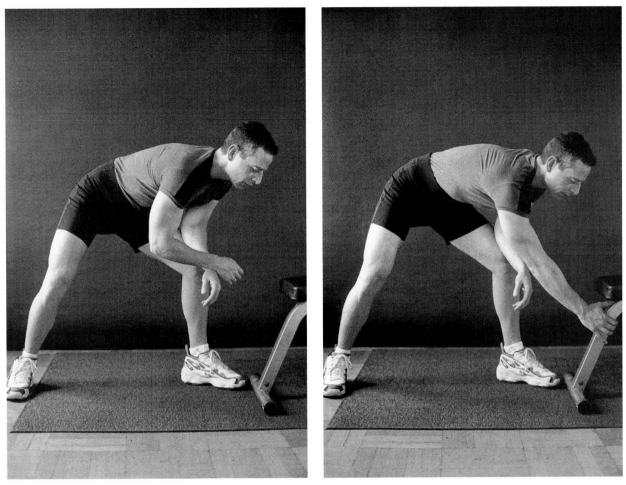

Figure 5.42*a*  Lat Stretch.

Figure 5.42*b*

## EXERCISE 42  LAT STRETCH
*Upper and middle back*

With this movement, you'll need something to grab onto, such as a heavy piece of furniture or a machine. Stand with feet slightly wider than shoulder width in a boxer's stance, left foot forward. *Exhale* and bend at the waist (Figure 5.42*a*), grabbing your anchor at about three feet above floor level with your right hand. Lean away from the object you're holding onto, and breathe into the movement (Figure 5.42*b*). *Inhale* as you let go. Repeat on the left.

*Hold time:*  15 to 30 seconds

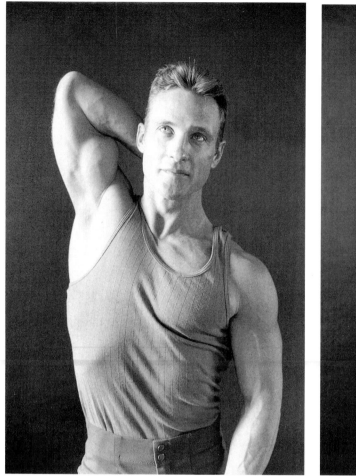

Figure 5.43*a*    Triceps Stretch.

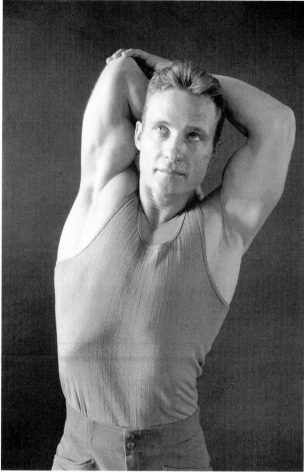

Figure 5.43*b*

## EXERCISE 43    TRICEPS STRETCH
*Triceps and shoulder*

Stand or sit and place your right arm over the top of your head, elbow bent (Figure 5.43*a*). Place your left hand on the back of your right elbow, *exhale*, and press, feeling a stretch in the back of your right arm (Figure 5.43*b*). Breathe and hold. *Inhale* as you release. Repeat with the left arm.

*Hold time:*  15 to 30 seconds

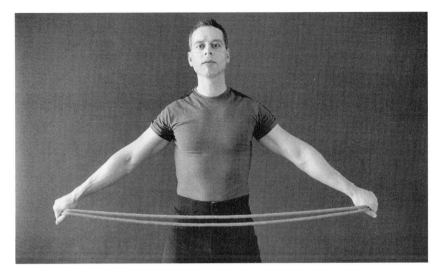

Figure 5.44*a*

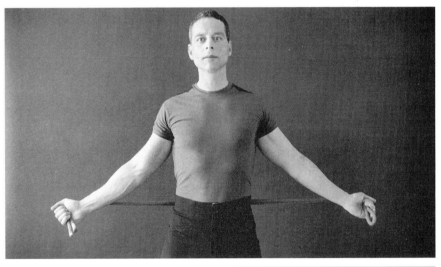

Figure 5.44*b*    Pullover Stretch
with Rope.

## EXERCISE 44    PULLOVER STRETCH WITH ROPE

*Shoulders and upper back*

For this movement, you'll need a strap or rope approximately five feet long. Grasp the strap at each end with both your palms facing either forward or behind you (Figure 5.44*a*). Keeping your arms extended at your sides, rotate both arms over your head so the strap winds up behind you (Figure 5.44*b*). Coordinate breathing and repetitions, *inhaling* as you lift your arms overhead from front to back, and *exhaling* as you lift from back to front. This is a great move to cool down after a shoulder workout, keeping flexibility in the often-tight shoulder and upper-back muscles.

*Repetitions:* 10 to 20

## SECTION 5.3 ROUTINES

On the next few pages the routines are outlined and grouped together in proper order and sequence, presented from the simple to the complex. Also included are suggestions on when to include your cardiovascular training (see Chapter 3 for details). This can be on alternate days from your strength and flexibility workouts, or on the same day depending on your time restrictions and energy levels. A simple five-minute walk, jog, or bike ride serves as a warmup and precedes every resistance workout while the flexibility segment concludes it. Be sure to include some of the stretches after your aerobic training, as well (especially lower-body stretches).

### THE RULES

1. Warm up and cool down for *every* workout.
2. Rest from 48 to 96 hours between training sessions on the same muscle group.
3. Beginners should *never* do anything two days in a row, including *intense* aerobic work.
4. As a general rule, rest one to two minutes between sets unless otherwise indicated.
5. Be flexible in scheduling your workouts; the days presented here are suggestions. Feel free to adapt the program to fit your schedule. If you're not able to complete a full workout due to *time* or *energy* restrictions, remember that a partial workout is better than no workout. Do what you can and realize that tomorrow is another day.
6. Ideally, your aerobic training should be done on alternate days from your strength training, but if you only have three days a week to work out, combine the two.
7. Time-saving tip: Flexibility training should normally be done after the aerobic and/or strength-training segments, but to save time many of the stretches can be intermixed with strength exercises, provided your body has had a chance to warm up.
8. Beginners should start slowly and do only as much as they can handle, gradually building up. Let common sense prevail, and always err on the side of caution.
9. Vary your training program by switching to the alternate exercises presented with most of the movements. Changing things every two or three months prevents your body from becoming accustomed to your present training regimen. Other variables might include the amount of resistance used, the number of repetitions performed, the number of sets, and the length of time between sets. See Routines 5 and 6 for other ways of shocking the muscles into growth. After you find a program that suits you and you've adapted to it, feel free to make changes and modifications to meet your individual needs.
10. Rate and record your intensity level:

| | |
|---|---|
| 1 | No workout |
| 2 | No muscle fatigue experienced during the lift |
| 3 | Minor muscle fatigue experienced on the last repetition |
| 4 | Major muscle fatigue felt on the last few repetitions |
| 5 | Total muscle failure, unable to perform one more repetition with proper form |
| + | Halfway to next level |

**IMPORTANT NOTE:** Anyone embarking on an exercise program is advised to seek the advice of a health care professional and get a complete physical exam before beginning.

## ROUTINE 1
### Full-Body Routine (Routine 1a or Routine 1b; Beginner to Intermediate Level)

**Primary Goal: Increased Lean Muscle Mass**
*Suggested strength-training days:* Monday, Wednesday, and Friday (or three other nonconsecutive days)
*Suggested aerobic conditioning days:* Tuesday and Thursday (or two other nonconsecutive days)

**Primary Goal: Fat Loss**
*Suggested strength-training days:* Tuesday and Thursday (or two other nonconsecutive days)
*Suggested aerobic conditioning days:* Monday, Wednesday, and Friday (or three other nonconsecutive days)

**IMPORTANT NOTE:** If the full-body routine is repeated three times a week, it should be performed at a lower intensity level that's more suitable for a beginner. When reaching higher intensity levels, switch to the split routine or strength train only twice a week. See the 30-minute full-body routine (Routine 1a), or circuit training (Routine 3) for the fastest and most efficient strength and flexibility programs.

## ROUTINE 2
### Split Routine (Routine 2a and Routine 2b; Beginner to Intermediate Level)

**Primary Goal: Increased Lean Muscle Mass**
*Suggested Strength-Training Days:* Monday (Routine 2a), Tuesday (Routine 2b), Thursday (Routine 2a), and Friday (Routine 2b)
*Suggested aerobic conditioning days:* Wednesday and Saturday

**Primary Goal: Fat Loss**
*Suggested strength-training days:* Week 1—Monday (Routine 2a), Wednesday (Routine 2b), and Friday (Routine 2a); Week 2—Monday (Routine 2b), Wednesday (Routine 2a), and Friday (Routine 2b)
*Suggested aerobic conditioning days:* Tuesday, Thursday, and Saturday

**IMPORTANT NOTE:** The split routine can be performed at higher intensity levels than the full-body routine due to the longer rest periods between training of the same muscles or muscle groups.

# ROUTINE 1A    30-MINUTE FULL-BODY ROUTINE

## STRENGTH SEGMENT

| STRENGTH EXERCISE | ALTERNATE | MUSCLE GROUP | NUMBER OF SETS |
|---|---|---|---|
| Squats | Lunges | Legs, gluteus | 3 with warmup |
| Bench press | Push-ups | Chest, shoulders | 3 with warmup |
| Bent row | Pullover | Back | 3 with warmup |
| Lateral raise | Shoulder press | Shoulders | 3 with warmup |
| Sit-ups | Leg raises | Abdominals | 2 |

## FLEXIBILITY SEGMENT

| STRETCH | MUSCLE GROUP | SETS AND HOLD |
|---|---|---|
| Hamstring step stretch | Hamstring | 1 or 2; 15 to 30 seconds |
| Triangle stretch | Inner thigh | 1 or 2; 15 to 30 seconds |
| Star stretch | Lower Back, inner thigh | 1 or 2; 10 to 20 seconds |
| Bridge | Quad stretch, back flex | 1 or 2; 10 to 20 seconds |
| Knee-to-chest stretch | Lower back | 1 or 2; 5 to 30 seconds |
| Crossover stretch | Lower back | 1 or 2; 5 to 10 seconds |
| Chest stretch | Chest | 1 or 2; 15 to 30 seconds |
| Shoulder crossover | Shoulders | 1 or 2; 15 to 30 seconds |

# ROUTINE 1B    EXTENDED FULL-BODY ROUTINE

## STRENGTH SEGMENT

| STRENGTH EXERCISE | ALTERNATE | MUSCLE GROUP | NUMBER OF SETS |
|---|---|---|---|
| Squats | Lunges | Legs, gluteus | 3 with warmup |
| Step-ups | Standing kickback | Legs, gluteus | 3 with warmup |
| Standing calf raise | One-leg calf raise | Calves | 3 with warmup |
| Bench press | Push-ups | Chest, shoulders | 3 with warmup |
| Bent row | Pullover | Back | 3 with warmup |
| Lateral raise | Shoulder press | Shoulders | 3 with warmup |
| Seated curl | Standing curl | Biceps | 3 with warmup |
| Kickback | Bench dip | Triceps | 3 with warmup |
| Sit-ups | Leg raises | Abdominals | 2 |
| Bridge (flexibility section) | Reverse leg raises | Lower Back, gluteus | 2 |

## FLEXIBILITY SEGMENT

| STRETCH | MUSCLE GROUP | SETS AND HOLD |
|---|---|---|
| Step stretch | Hamstring | 1 or 2; 15 to 30 seconds |
| Triangle stretch | Inner thigh | 1 or 2; 15 to 30 seconds |
| Calf stretch | Calves | 1 or 2; 15 to 30 seconds |
| Star stretch | Lower back, inner thigh | 1 or 2; 10 to 20 seconds |
| Knee-to-chest stretch | Lower back | 1 or 2; 5 to 30 seconds |
| Crossover stretch | Lower back | 1 or 2; 5 to 10 seconds |
| Chest stretch | Chest | 1 or 2; 15 to 30 seconds |
| Shoulder crossover | Shoulders | 1 or 2; 15 to 30 seconds |
| Lat stretch | Back | 1 or 2; 15 to 30 seconds |
| Triceps stretch | Triceps | 1 or 2; 15 to 30 seconds |

*Note:* Warm up with a 5-minute walk, jog, or other exercise.

## ROUTINE 2A    SPLIT ROUTINE (LEGS, ARMS, AND CORE)

### STRENGTH SEGMENT

| STRENGTH EXERCISE | ALTERNATE | MUSCLE GROUP | NUMBER OF SETS |
|---|---|---|---|
| Squats | Lunges | Legs, gluteus | 3 or 4 with warmup |
| Step-ups | Standing kickback | Legs, gluteus | 3 with warmup |
| Standing calf raise | One-leg calf raise | Calves | 3 with warmup |
| Seated curl | Standing curl | Biceps | 3 with warmup |
| Triceps press | Kickback | Triceps | 3 with warmup |
| Sit-ups | Leg raises | Abdominal | 2 |
| Reverse leg raise | Bridge (flexibility section) | Lower back, gluteus | 2 |
| Side leg raise | | Oblique | 2 |

### FLEXIBILITY SEGMENT

| STRETCH | MUSCLE GROUP | SETS AND HOLD |
|---|---|---|
| Step stretch | Hamstring | 1 or 2; 15 to 30 seconds |
| Triangle stretch | Inner thigh | 1 or 2; 15 to 30 seconds |
| Calf stretch | Calves | 1 or 2; 15 to 30 seconds |
| Star stretch | Lower back, inner thigh | 1 or 2; 10 to 20 seconds |
| Bridge | Quad stretch, back flex | 1 or 2; 5 to 20 seconds |
| Alternate leg stretch | Hamstring | 1 or 2; 15 to 30 seconds |
| Knee-to-chest stretch | Lower back | 1 or 2; 5 to 30 seconds |
| Crossover stretch | Lower back | 1 or 2; 5 to 10 seconds |
| Triceps stretch | Triceps | 1 or 2; 15 to 30 seconds |

## ROUTINE 2B    SPLIT ROUTINE (CHEST, BACK, AND SHOULDERS)

### STRENGTH SEGMENT

| STRENGTH EXERCISE | ALTERNATE | MUSCLE GROUP | NUMBER OF SETS |
|---|---|---|---|
| Bench press | Incline press | Chest, shoulders | 3 or 4 with warmup |
| Incline press | Fly | Chest, shoulders | 3 with warmup |
| Cable row | Bent row | Back | 3 or 4 with warmup |
| Bent row | Pullovers | Back | 3 with warmup |
| Lateral raise | Shoulder press | Shoulders | 3 with warmup |
| Rear lateral raise | Upright row | Shoulders (rear) | 3 with warmup |

### FLEXIBILITY SEGMENT

| STRETCH | MUSCLE GROUP | SETS AND HOLD |
|---|---|---|
| Step stretch | Hamstring | 1 or 2; 15 to 30 seconds |
| Star stretch | Lower back, inner thigh | 1 or 2; 10 to 20 seconds |
| Bridge | Quad stretch, back flex | 1 or 2; 5 to 20 seconds |
| Knee-to-chest stretch | Lower back | 1 or 2; 5 to 30 seconds |
| Crossover stretch | Lower back | 1 or 2; 5 to 10 seconds |
| Chest stretch | Chest | 1 or 2; 15 to 30 seconds |
| Shoulder crossover | Shoulders | 1 or 2; 15 to 30 seconds |
| Lat stretch | Back | 1 or 2; 15 to 30 seconds |
| Triceps stretch | Triceps | 1 or 2; 15 to 30 seconds |

*Note:* Warm up with a 5-minute walk, jog, or other exercise.

## ROUTINE 3
### Full-Body Circuit Training
### (Intermediate Level; Fast and Efficient)

**Primary Goal: Balance of Increased Lean Muscle Mass and Fat Loss**

*Suggested strength-training days:* Tuesday and Thursday (or two other nonconsecutive days)

*Suggested aerobic conditioning days:* Monday, Wednesday, and Friday (or three other nonconsecutive days)

**IMPORTANT NOTE:** This circuit has two distinct segments: (1) lower body and core and (2) upper body.

▶ No rest time is permitted within each part.

▶ Rest three minutes between each segment of the circuit.

▶ Perform the entire routine before repeating.

▶ Be prepared to use lighter weight than when not circuit training.

▶ This routine can be applied to all or any portion of your strength workout.

▶ Circuit training can also be done as a *split routine* four times a week: Segment 3*a*—lower body and core; Segment 3*b*—upper body.

## ROUTINE 4
### Maintenance Program
### (Intermediate Level)

**Primary Goal: Maintenance of Lean Muscle Mass**

*Suggested strength-training days:* Monday, Wednesday, and Friday (or two or three other nonconsecutive days)

*Suggested aerobic conditioning days:* Tuesday, Thursday, and Saturday (or two or three other nonconsecutive days)

**IMPORTANT NOTE:** The entire maintenance program can be performed two or three days a week. It can also be performed as a split routine four days a week or be combined with your cardiovascular training. It can be used as an *active rest* workout following lengthy cycles of intense training.

## STRENGTH SEGMENT

| STRENGTH EXERCISE | ALTERNATE | MUSCLE GROUP |
|---|---|---|
| **SEGMENT 3A (LOWER BODY AND CORE)** | | |
| Squat | Lunges | Legs, gluteus |
| Standing kickback | Step-ups | Legs, gluteus |
| Calf raise | One leg calf raise | Calves |
| Leg raises | Sit-ups | Abdominals |
| Reverse leg raises | Bridge (flex. sec.) | Lower back, gluteus |
| **SEGMENT 3B (UPPER BODY)*** | | |
| Bench press | Fly | Chest, shoulders |
| Cable row | Bent row | Back |
| Lateral raise | Shoulder press | Shoulders |
| Standing curl | Concentration curl | Biceps |
| Triceps press | Kickback | Triceps |

## FLEXIBILITY SEGMENT

| STRETCH | MUSCLE GROUP | SETS AND HOLD |
|---|---|---|
| Step stretch | Hamstring | 1 or 2; 15 to 30 seconds |
| Triangle stretch | Inner thigh | 1 or 2; 15 to 30 seconds |
| Calf stretch | Calves | 1 or 2; 15 to 30 seconds |
| Star stretch | Lower back, inner thigh | 1 or 2; 10 to 20 seconds |
| Bridge | Quad stretch, back flex | 1 or 2; 5 to 20 seconds |
| Alternate leg stretch | Hamstring | 1 or 2; 15 to 30 seconds |
| Knee-to-chest stretch | Lower back | 1 or 2; 5 to 30 seconds |
| Crossover stretch | Lower back | 1 or 2; 5 to 10 seconds |
| Chest stretch | Chest | 1 or 2; 15 to 30 seconds |
| Shoulder crossover | Shoulders | 1 or 2; 15 to 30 seconds |
| Lat stretch | Back | 1 or 2; 15 to 30 seconds |
| Triceps stretch | Triceps | 1 or 2; 15 to 30 seconds |

*Note:* Warm up with a 5-minute walk, jog, or other exercise.

*Rest 3 minutes between segments. Repeat the entire routine two or three times depending on your level of fitness.

## STRENGTH SEGMENT

| STRENGTH EXERCISE | ALTERNATE | MUSCLE GROUP | NUMBER OF SETS |
| --- | --- | --- | --- |
| Squats | Lunges | Legs, glutes | 3 with warmup |
| Calf raise | One-leg calf raise | Calves | 3 with warmup |
| Bench press | Incline press | Chest, shoulders | 3 with warmup |
| Cable row | Bent row | Back | 3 with warmup |
| Shoulder press | Lateral raise | Shoulders | 3 with warmup |
| Standing curl | Seated curl | Biceps | 2 or 3 with warmup |
| Triceps press | Bench dip | Triceps | 2 or 3 with warmup |
| Sit-ups | Leg raises | Abdominals | 1 or 2 |

## FLEXIBILITY SEGMENT

| STRETCH | MUSCLE GROUP | SETS AND HOLD |
| --- | --- | --- |
| Step stretch | Hamstring | 1 or 2; 15 to 30 seconds |
| Triangle stretch | Inner thigh | 1 or 2; 15 to 30 seconds |
| Calf stretch | Calves | 1 or 2; 15 to 30 seconds |
| Star stretch | Lower back, inner thigh | 1 or 2; 10 to 20 seconds |
| Bridge | Quad stretch, back flex | 1 or 2; 5 to 20 seconds |
| Alternate leg stretch | Hamstring | 1 or 2; 15 to 30 seconds |
| Knee-to-chest stretch | Lower back | 1 or 2; 5 to 30 seconds |
| Crossover stretch | Lower back | 1 or 2; 5 to 10 seconds |
| Chest stretch | Chest | 1 or 2; 15 to 30 seconds |
| Shoulder crossover | Shoulders | 1 or 2; 15 to 30 seconds |
| Lat stretch | Back | 1 or 2; 15 to 30 seconds |
| Triceps stretch | Triceps | 1 or 2; 15 to 30 seconds |

*Note:* Warm up with a 5-minute walk, jog, or other exercise.

**ROUTINE 5**
**Pyramid Training**
**(Intermediate to Advanced Level)**

**Primary Goal: Increased Lean Muscle Mass**
Pyramid training can be applied to Routines 1, 2, and 4 or any portion thereof. Apply the following to any exercise:

*Set 1.* Perform one warmup set for 20 reps.

*Set 2.* Increase the weight so that you can complete 12 to 15 reps to muscle fatigue.

*Set 3.* Increase the weight so that you can complete 8 to 10 reps to muscle fatigue.

*Set 4.* Increase the weight so that you can complete 6 to 8 reps to muscle fatigue or *failure*.

*Set 5 (optional).* *Decrease* the weight to that of Set 2 or 3 and lift to muscle fatigue or *failure* regardless of the number of reps. This set can be performed with no rest, but allow normal rest (1 to 2 minutes) between all other sets.

**IMPORTANT NOTE:** Pyramid training allows you to increase intensity levels, and is a great way to shock the muscles into further growth.

**ROUTINE 6**
**Slow-Motion Training**
**(Intermediate to Advanced Level)**

**Primary Goal: Increased Lean Muscle Mass**
Slow-motion training can be applied to Routines 1, 2, 3, or 4 or any portion thereof. Select a weight that's light enough for you to execute the following:

*Positive phase.* On the positive or up phase of each rep, lift to a slow count of 4 with perfect form and no cheating whatsoever.

*Negative phase.* On the negative or down phase of the lift, lower to a slow count of 8, controlling the weight as you lower it against gravity.

**IMPORTANT NOTE:** Slow-motion training is an excellent way to increase intensity without using heavier weight.

The exercises presented here have mostly been demonstrated with minimal equipment but can be easily adapted to more sophisticated machines. The basic principles remain the same and should always be adhered to. The sample exercise records at the end of the chapter show routines over a three-day period.

## FIGURE 5.45   DAILY EXERCISE RECORD

**Strength Routine**      **Full Body**                          **Joe Cool    1/1/00**

| WARMUP | MODE: | TM | | DURATION: | | 5 | |
|---|---|---|---|---|---|---|---|

| MUSCLE GROUP | EXERCISE | SET 1 | SET 2 | SET 3 | SET 4 | SET 5 | COMMENTS |
|---|---|---|---|---|---|---|---|
| | | | | WEIGHT/REPETITIONS | | | |
| Legs | Squats BB | 40/20 | 60/15 | 80/12 | 90/8 | | Use the comments |
| | Step-ups DB | 20/20 | 20/20 | 30/15 | | | section to record |
| | Calf raises | /20 | /20 | | | | your intensity |
| | | | | | | | levels or include |
| Chest | Bench press DB | 20/20 | 30/30 | 30/12 | | | as a third column. |
| | | | | | | | 30/15/4 |
| Back | Rows DB | 20/20 | 30/16 | 35/10 | | | 4 |
| Shoulders | Lateral raises DB | 5/20 | 10/15 | 10/12 | | | 5 |
| Arms/biceps | Seated curl DB | 15/20 | 30/12 | | | | 4 |
| Arms/triceps | Kickbacks DB | 10/20 | 15/15 | 15/12 | | | 4 |

**Flexibility Routine**      **Full body**

| MUSCLE GROUP | EXERCISE | SET 1 | SET 2 | SET 3 | SET 4 | SET 5 | COMMENTS |
|---|---|---|---|---|---|---|---|
| | | INDICATE A CHECK OR HOLD TIME FOR EACH SET COMPLETED | | | | | |
| Step stretch | Hamstring | 15 | 15 | 15 | | | Feeling tight today. |
| Triangle | Inner thigh | 15 | 15 | | | | Looking forward to |
| Calf | Calf | 30 | | | | | next workout. |
| Star | Low back & thigh | 10 | 10 | 10 | | | |
| Knee to chest | Low back | 5 | 5 | 5 | | | |
| Crossover | Low back | 5 | 5 | 5 | | | |
| Chest exp | Chest | 15 | 15 | | | | |
| Shldr cross | Shoulders | 15 | 15 | | | | |
| Back stretch | Back | 15 | 15 | | | | |
| Triceps stretch | Triceps | 15 | 15 | | | | |

| CARDIO ROUTINE | MODE | DURATION | MAX HEART RATE | COMMENTS |
|---|---|---|---|---|
| | | | | Cardio rest today. |

## FIGURE 5.47  DAILY EXERCISE RECORD

**Strength Routine**                              **Joe Cool   1/2/00**

| WARMUP | MODE: | TM | DURATION: | 5 | | | |
|--------|-------|-----|-----------|-----|-----|-----|-----|
| **MUSCLE GROUP** | **EXERCISE** | **SET 1** | **SET 2** | **SET 3** | **SET 4** | **SET 5** | **COMMENTS** |
| **WEIGHT/REPETITIONS** | | | | | | | |
| | | | | | | | |
| | | | | | | | |
| | | | | | | | |
| | | | | | | | |
| | | | | | | | |

**Flexibility Routine**      **Full body**

| MUSCLE GROUP | EXERCISE | SET 1 | SET 2 | SET 3 | SET 4 | SET 5 | COMMENTS |
|--------------|----------|-------|-------|-------|-------|-------|----------|
| **INDICATE A CHECK OR HOLD TIME FOR EACH SET COMPLETED** | | | | | | | |
| Step stretch | Hamstring | 15 | 15 | 15 | | | Starting to open up. |
| Triangle | Inner thigh | 15 | 15 | | | | |
| Calf | Calf | 30 | | | | | |
| Star | Low back & thigh | 10 | 10 | 10 | | | |
| Knee to chest | Low back | 5 | 5 | 5 | | | |
| Crossover | Low back | 5 | 5 | 5 | | | |
| Chest exp | Chest | 15 | 15 | | | | |
| Shldr cross | Shoulders | 15 | 15 | | | | |
| Back stretch | Back | 15 | 15 | | | | |
| Triceps stretch | Triceps | 15 | 15 | | | | |

| **Cardio Routine** | **Mode** | **Duration** | **Max Heart Rate** | **Comments** |
|---------------------|----------|--------------|---------------------|---------------|
| | Running | 30 | 150 | Felt tired today. |

## FIGURE 5.46  DAILY EXERCISE RECORD

**Strength Routine**    **Full Body**                    Joe Cool   1/3/00

| WARMUP | MODE: | TM | DURATION: | | 5 | | |
|---|---|---|---|---|---|---|---|
| **MUSCLE GROUP** | **EXERCISE** | **SET 1** | **SET 2** | **SET 3** | **SET 4** | **SET 5** | **COMMENTS** |
| | | **WEIGHT/REPETITIONS** | | | | | |
| Legs | Squats BB | 40/20 | 60/15 | 80/12 | 90/8 | | Use the comments |
| | Step-ups DB | 20/20 | 20/20 | 30/15 | | | section to record |
| | Calf raises | /20 | /20 | | | | your intensity |
| | | | | | | | levels or include |
| Chest | Bench press DB | 20/20 | 30/30 | 30/12 | | | as a third column. |
| | | | | | | | 30/15/4 |
| Back | Rows DB | 20/20 | 30/16 | 35/10 | | | 4 |
| Shoulders | Lateral raises DB | 5/20 | 10/15 | 10/12 | | | 5 |
| Arms/biceps | Seated curl DB | 15/20 | 30/12 | | | | 4 |
| Arms/triceps | Kickbacks DB | 10/20 | 15/15 | 15/12 | | | 4 |

**Flexibility Routine**    **Full body**

| MUSCLE GROUP | EXERCISE | SET 1 | SET 2 | SET 3 | SET 4 | SET 5 | COMMENTS |
|---|---|---|---|---|---|---|---|
| | | **INDICATE A CHECK OR HOLD TIME FOR EACH SET COMPLETED** | | | | | |
| Step stretch | Hamstring | 15 | 15 | 15 | | | Feeling tight today. |
| Triangle | Inner thigh | 15 | 15 | | | | Looking forward to |
| Calf | Calf | 30 | | | | | next workout. |
| Star | Low back & thigh | 10 | 10 | 10 | | | |
| Knee to Chest | Low back | 5 | 5 | 5 | | | |
| Crossover | Low back | 5 | 5 | 5 | | | |
| Chest exp | Chest | 15 | 15 | | | | |
| Shldr cross | Shoulders | 15 | 15 | | | | |
| Back stretch | Back | 15 | 15 | | | | |
| Triceps stretch | Triceps | 15 | 15 | | | | |

| Cardio Routine | Mode | Duration | Max Heart Rate | Comments |
|---|---|---|---|---|
| | Running | 30 | 150 | Felt strong today. |

# THE SHIRT

The loose-fitting station uniform concealed any muscle-mass gains I'd made over the past couple of years until the night I wore a tight-fitting athletic T-shirt. I'd been training pretty hard, applying the principles and practices of the Firefighter's Workout to myself, and getting fantastic results.

It was a warm summer evening in New York City when the crew and I decided to relieve some stress with a night out. I showered and quickly dressed in front of my metal locker. Pulling the shirt over my head, I trotted down the stairs to the sitting room.

When I walked through the door they were ready for me. "Hey Cap, is that your sister's shirt you're wearing?" was followed quickly by "Did we miss the Kids 'R' Us sale last week?" They had noticed the muscle gains the baggy uniform had concealed during the past two years, which my tight shirt now revealed. I smiled to myself and answered, "No, she got this one at The Gap."

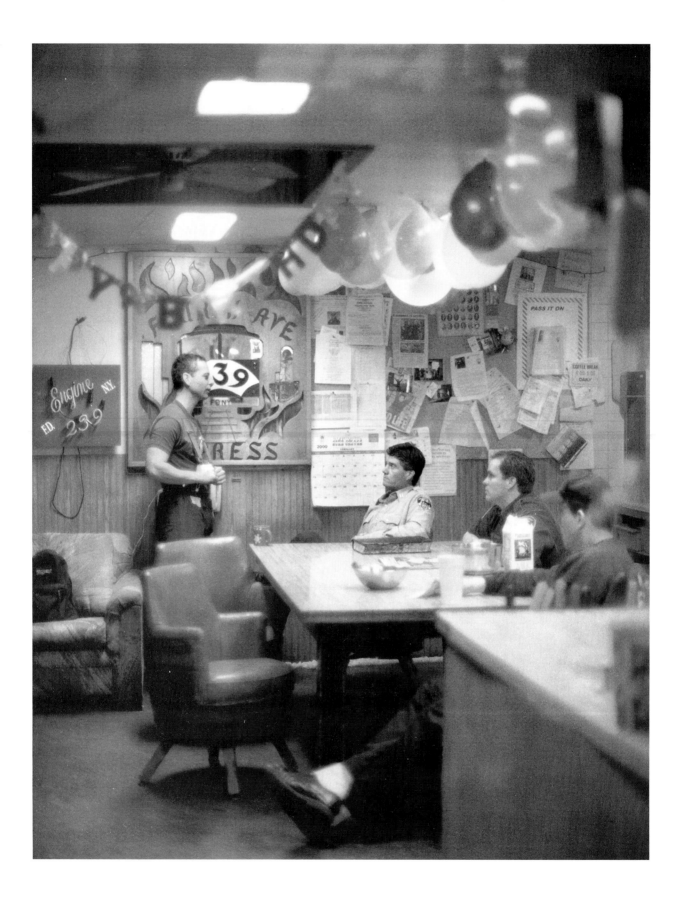

# CHAPTER SIX

# Evaluating Your Program

**A**t the scene of any major fire, the chief in charge has to make frequent progress reports to the fire department's central command. These progress reports reveal whether the tactics being applied are working. They also tell central command whether the firefighters and resources on the scene are being overtaxed or underutilized, or whether any adjustments need to be made.

The same theory holds for your fitness program. Pay close attention to what works best and what doesn't work so well. Just as each fire or emergency operation is handled differently, each person is unique in his or her exercise and nutritional needs.

In order to accurately track your progress, you have to record the results of the initial *fitness assessment* as well as recording all of your workouts. Include some comments and observations on each workout session. In this way, your workout records will also serve as a fitness diary or a daily commentary on your training program. Sample fitness assessment charts for a man and a woman appear in this section. Blank charts for recording both your daily training sessions and your fitness assessment are in Appendix C.

## SECTION 6.1   FITNESS ASSESSMENT

**T**his is not about comparison but rather measuring progress as a way to ensure the best possible training program. This section presents six *fitness assessment tests.* You can choose to take them or not. There is no rating, but their simplicity makes them very easy to accomplish. I also recommend taking a photo of yourself and filing it away with your initial assessment chart. A picture is worth a thousand words (or, in this case, numbers). Health clubs in your area may offer free fitness assessments in an effort to attract more clientele. I encourage you to take advantage of any such offer even if you don't join.

*Make sure you warm up before Tests 1, 2, and 3.*

1. *Push-up test (upper-body strength and endurance).* Perform as many push-ups (see Chapter 5) or modified push-ups as you can with proper form and record the number.
2. *Step test (lower-body and cardiorespiratory endurance).* Set up a workout step with a height of 12

inches. Step up and down with alternating feet at a pace of 96 beats per minute (a digital metronome or stop watch can be purchased rather cheaply at your local sporting goods store, or estimate three steps every two seconds) for three minutes. Immediately afterward, monitor your pulse rate for one full minute and record.

3. *Sit-and-reach test (upper-and lower-body flexibility).* Sit on the floor, legs straight out in front of you, back straight. Place a tape measure between your legs with the 15-inch mark at your heel, the numbers increasing as they go away from you. Reach out and down as far as you can. Record the inch mark where the tips of your fingers reach the tape.

4. *Circumference measurements.* Take circumference measurements of your waist, hips, chest, thighs, and upper arms with a standard tape measure and record.

5. *Body weight.* Record your present body weight in pounds.

6. *Body-fat composition.* There are many ways to measure body fat, including the following:

   ▶ *Hydrostatic weighing.* Accurate but expensive and impractical.

   ▶ *Bioelectric impedance.* As reliable as the skin-fold method.

   ▶ *Body mass index.* Divide weight (kilograms) by height (meters) squared.

   ▶ *Skin-fold measurements.* Valid, reliable, inexpensive, and convenient.

   The skin-fold measurement method will give you a reasonable and reliable estimation of your body-fat percentages. A *body-fat caliper* can be purchased for as little as $10 and used safely and conveniently in the privacy of your own home. Simply follow the instruction booklet that comes with the caliper and record your results. Here are some additional considerations:

   ▶ All measurements are taken on the right side of the body.

▶ Grasp the skin fold firmly with the thumb and index finger of the left hand.

▶ Hold the caliper perpendicular to the site.

▶ Maintain the pads approximately a quarter inch from the thumb and index finger.

▶ Add results; look up percentage on the proper chart and record.

Here are some common sites for skin-fold measurement:

**MEN**

▶ Chest—diagonal skinfold midway on the crease of underarm and nipple

▶ Abdomen—vertical fold one inch to the right of the navel

▶ Thigh—vertical fold midway between the hip and the knee

**WOMEN**

▶ Triceps—vertical fold on the back of the upper arm between the shoulder and elbow

▶ Hip—diagonal fold at the crest of the hip bone

▶ Thigh—vertical fold midway between the hip and the knee

## BODY-FAT PERCENTAGE LEVELS

| CLASSIFICATION | WOMEN | MEN |
| --- | --- | --- |
| Essential fat | 10–12 | 2–4 |
| Athlete | 14–20 | 6–13 |
| Fit | 21–24 | 14–17 |
| Acceptable | 25–31 | 18–25 |
| Obese | 32 and higher | 25 and higher |

After your initial fitness assessment, I suggest reassessment at three-month intervals. In addition to assessments, pay attention to the progress you're making in your workouts, as well as to how you look and feel. At the beginning of an exercise program, you should expect gradual but steady progress.

**STRENGTH-TRAINING PROGRAM**

▶ Are you seeing a gradual increase in the amount of weight you're able to lift or the number of repetitions you're able to complete?

▶ Do you see or feel an increase in terms of muscle mass?

**CARDIOVASCULAR CONDITIONING PROGRAM**

▶ Are you able to perform at a faster pace or for a longer duration with succeeding workouts?

▶ Are you leaner, or are your clothes fitting differently?

**FLEXIBILITY PROGRAM**

▶ Are you becoming more limber and able to stretch further?

▶ Do you feel less tense, especially in the neck and lower-back areas?

Your program should enable you to answer yes to at least some of these questions. If not, something in your exercise or nutritional program is lacking and needs to be addressed. Performing fitness assessments and monitoring your workouts will enable you to make the necessary adjustments to achieve success.

---

## SECTION 6.2  REST AND RECUPERATION

Quick recovery is a vital ingredient of the Firefighter's Workout. An exercise or nutritional program that left you wiped out and unable to perform at full capacity might become a liability to any working firefighter. In this section, we'll go over some additional safeguards to help you avoid any problems related to excessive training.

## Overtraining

So far, we have not made much mention of overtraining. The Firefighter's Workout makes it particularly difficult to overtrain, *if* you stick to the guidelines. There will always be overzealous exercisers who'll take it a step further—some of them will be able to handle it, some will not.

For most people, overtraining (or training too much) will prove counterproductive. You'll get sick, feel tired, risk an overuse injury, and suffer a host of other nasty symptoms. It's your body's way of telling you to slow down. Listen to your body and either take a week or two completely off or ease up on the duration, frequency, and intensity of your workouts. If it's rest your body needs, allow yourself to have it.

If you experience any pain that doesn't go away in a few days, stop all exercise and see a physician as soon as possible.

## The Sleep Factor

New York City firefighters (as well as most firefighters across the country) are required to work long shifts, sometimes 24 hours at a time. This often translates into an overall lack of sleep, which they must compensate for by easing up on their workout programs.

There is no doubt that exercise increases the need for fit, restful sleep. The good news is that it also increases your ability to sleep soundly. Individual sleep requirements differ, but most people need about seven or eight hours of sound sleep nightly. During sleep the body repairs and replenishes itself and gets stronger, and sleep is a vital ingredient in the success of any exercise program.

## A Word to Seniors

I'm a firm believer that people of any age can benefit from a fitness program, but with time the body's ability to repair itself slows somewhat. You have to make necessary adjustments to avoid injury and continue to improve. You may have to decrease the frequency, duration, and intensity of your program to allow your body to bounce back. Diet and sleep become vital in maintaining energy levels and the body's repair mechanisms. Men above the age of 40 and women above 50 should seek the advice of a physician before beginning.

## Other Risk Factors

Anyone embarking upon an exercise program should seek the advice of a health care professional before starting. There are certain risk factors that make this mandatory. If you fall into any of the following categories, see a doctor and get a complete physical exam before you begin.

▶ Age (men over 40, women over 50)
▶ Smoking
▶ Heart disease
▶ High serum cholesterol level ($\geq$200 mg/dl)
▶ Diabetes mellitus
▶ High blood pressure (>140 over 90 mm Hg)
▶ Sedentary lifestyle
▶ Family history of heart disease

# FITNESS ASSESSMENT

**Joe Cool**

| FITNESS TEST | DATE 1/1/00 | DATE 4/1/00 | DATE 7/1/00 |
|---|---|---|---|
| Max push-up test | 22 | 24 | 30 |
| 3-minute step test | 102 | 100 | 96 |
| Sit-and-reach test | 13 | 15 | 17 |

| BODY COMPOSITION | DATE 1/1/00 | DATE 4/1/00 | DATE 7/1/00 |
|---|---|---|---|

Circumference Measurements

| | | | |
|---|---|---|---|
| Upper arm | 14 | 14½ | 15 |
| Thigh | 22 | 23 | 23 |
| Waist | 33 | 32 | 31 |
| Hips | 36 | 35 | 35 |
| Chest | 40 | 41 | 42 |
| | | | |
| Body Weight | 180 | 176 | 174 |

## BODY-FAT PERCENTAGE

| Method | Skin caliper | Skin caliper | Skin caliper |
|---|---|---|---|
| Percentage | 15 | 13 | 12 |

| PHYSICIAN'S SECTION | DATE 1/2/00 | DATE 4/1/00 | DATE 7/1/00 |
|---|---|---|---|
| Resting heart rate | 66 | 64 | 62 |
| Max heart rate | 175 | 175 | 175 |
| Blood pressure | 130/76 | 130/70 | 120/70 |
| Cholesterol level | 180 | 160 | 150 |
| Triglyceride level | 180 | 160 | 100 |

## FITNESS ASSESSMENT

**Jane Cool**

| FITNESS TEST | DATE 1/1/00 | DATE 4/1/00 | DATE 7/1/00 |
|---|---|---|---|
| Max push-up test | 16 | 18 | 22 |
| 3-minute step test | 110 | 100 | 96 |
| Sit-and-reach test | 16 | 17 | 18 |
| **BODY COMPOSITION** | DATE 1/1/00 | DATE 4/1/00 | DATE 7/1/00 |
| Circumference Measurements | | | |
| Upper arm | 11 | 11 | 12 |
| Thigh | 22 | 21 | 20 |
| Waist | 29 | 28 | 27 |
| Hips | 38 | 37 | 36 |
| Chest | 36 | 36 | 35 |
| | | | |
| Body Weight | 140 | 136 | 130 |

| BODY-FAT PERCENTAGE | | | |
|---|---|---|---|
| Method | Skin caliper | Skin caliper | Skin caliper |
| Percentage | 22 | 20 | 18 |
| **PHYSICIAN'S SECTION** | DATE 1/1/00 | DATE 4/1/00 | DATE 7/1/00 |
| Resting heart rate | 68 | 66 | 64 |
| Max heart rate | 190 | 190 | 190 |
| Blood pressure | 130/80 | 120/80 | 120/70 |
| Cholesterol level | 180 | 170 | 160 |
| Triglyceride level | 170 | 100 | 80 |

# BED STUY

Smoke permeated every inch of that tenement-lined Brooklyn street. At first, I thought we had a couple of cars burning in a parking lot at street level until I heard the desperate cries for help. The muffled screams were coming from a top-floor fire escape balcony as two terrified, sobbing children and their panicky baby-sitter hunched under the dense, heated black smoke that pushed out from the windows of their apartment.

I made my way into the building and two-stepped it up the six flights of stairs as the rest of my crew started the long arduous task of dragging 500 feet of high-pressure hose up the same six flights. When I got onto the fire floor landing, the hall went black with smoke. Instinctively, I dropped to my knees where the cooler, cleaner air still lingered. At floor level, I was able to see a long, narrow hall that seemed to go on forever. The crackling noises of the blaze served as my homing device, leading me in the right direction.

Once inside the apartment, I could see the hot orange flame lapping out of a back bedroom, cutting off the normal exit as it vented itself out the windows to the balcony the kids were on. I slithered under the fire rolling along the ceiling and reached the desperate trio.

That particular type of fire escape was intended to provide a path of escape, in the event of fire, to an adjoining fire-resistant apartment on the same floor. That night the path was blocked. One of the tenants apparently had seen fit to squeeze an oversized, dirt-filled flowerpot onto the narrow balcony, successfully sealing off any chance of someone going from apartment to apartment.

As the fire grew in intensity, conditions in the apartment and on the fire escape deteriorated rapidly. Thick, blinding smoke enveloped us, but the only way out was over, around, or through that massive flowerpot. I rocked, pushed, tugged, and pried. At first the huge pot didn't budge. I reached down, dug in, and thrust for all I was worth and managed to move it only a few inches, but those few inches were enough. Choking and gasping for air, all three squeezed through to the clean air of the adjoining apartment.

By this time, I heard the rest of my crew at the fire apartment door with their hose lines gushing with precious water, and I crawled back in to meet them. It was time to finish the job and slay the red devil that had almost taken the lives of three more innocent victims.

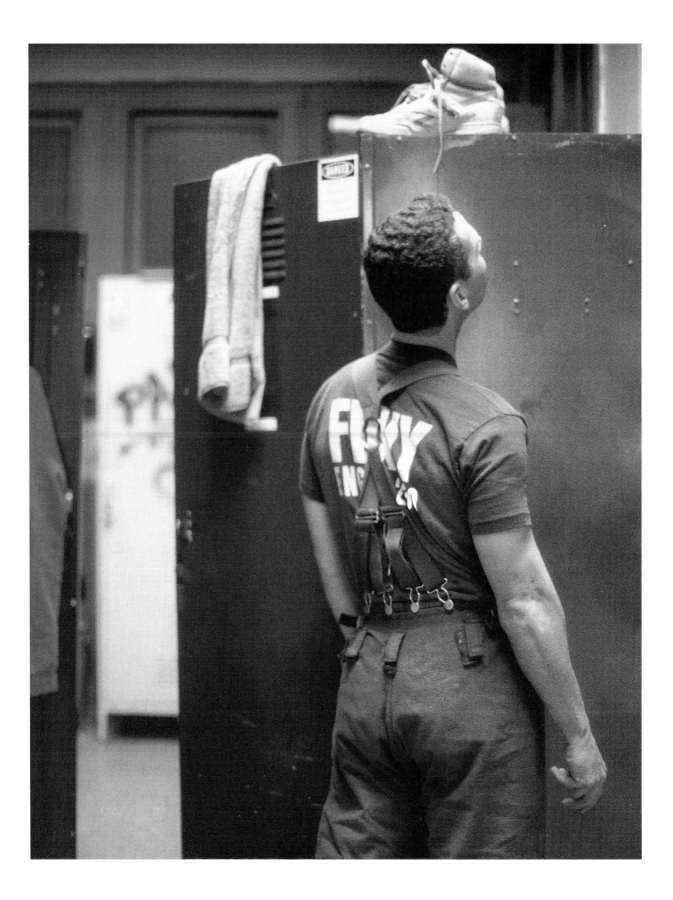

# Frequently Asked Questions

**O**ver the years I think I've heard every question on diet and exercise in the book. This section lists some of the most common, which I hope will answer any questions that may arise as you begin to train.

**Q:** *I'm a busy professional and don't have time to get to the gym every day. I live in a small apartment where I can't fit much exercise equipment. How can I maintain an exercise program that works?*

**A:** Go to the gym when you can but realize it's not necessary to use fancy health club machines to get the results you want. In order to save some time, work out at home. For a little over $100 dollars you can purchase a set of dumbbells and an athletic step which can serve as your bench, all of which can slide under a bed for hideaway storage. You'll only require a good pair of running or walking shoes to perform your cardio work, and you can stretch anywhere. The time you'll save traveling to and from the gym can be spent training.

**Q:** *What is the minimum amount of time I can spend training and still see good results?*

**A:** Of course, each of us responds differently to exercise, but in general you need to repeat strength training of a particular body part every 96 hours or less to continue to make progress. I suggest a *full-body routine* (see Chapter 5, Routine 1*a* or 1*b*) twice a week. Cut back on the number of sets or *circuit train* (see Chapter 5, Routine 3) to save more time, but do at least two sets of each exercise as a minimum. Cardio work needs to be done at least twice a week as well, and benefits can be seen with 15- or 20-minute workouts. Keep intensity levels high to ensure progress. Flexibility segments can be done with both strength and cardio work. Your nutrition program comes heavily into play with any type of workout program, but this becomes more evident when you cut corners on the length or number of training sessions.

**Q:** *I get bored doing the same movements, the same exercises, day in and day out. How can I avoid this boredom?*

**A:** Change the movements. I recommend changing your routines around every month or so. There are an infinite number of ways to accomplish this, and you can manipulate your workouts any way you like. You can change actual exercises by selecting alternate movements. You can also alter the weight lifted and thereby reduce or increase the number of repetitions performed. Do more sets, or fewer sets. Apply the variations found in Chapter 5, Routines 5 and 6.

Your cardio workout can consist of a different movement every time you do it as long as it gets you into the target heart-rate zone. Run today, bike tomorrow. It doesn't matter. Go out and play racquetball for an hour. This is about variety and enjoyment, not just hard work and discipline.

**Q:** *When is the best time for me to train?*

**A:** Any time you can. The bottom line is, work out when it's best and most convenient for you, increasing your chances of exercising more often. It's important to know in advance when those times will be and to stick to the schedule you make for yourself.

**Q:** *I train and train and train, but I can't seem to lose those last few pounds of fat around my midsection. What do I need to do?*

**A:** If you're satisfied with your exercise program and you still can't drop the pounds, try taking a closer look at your nutritional program. How many calories and grams of fat and sugar are you ingesting every day? Try switching to lower-calorie, more nutritionally dense foods, as explained in Chapter 4.

**Q:** *I'd like to put on about 5 or 10 pounds of muscle. What's the best way to accomplish this?*

**A:** Some find it hard to believe, but there are people out there who'd like to gain weight. Of course, the emphasis in your routine would be on strength training, keeping cardio work to a minimum. Do more sets with very low repetitions, adding weight each set (*pyramid training;* see Chapter 5, Routine 5), completing anywhere from four to eight reps on the last set. Keep intensity levels high, and allow ample time for recovery between sets as well as between workouts.

**Q:** *I'm training for the New York City Marathon. Should I still be strength training?*

**A:** Absolutely. Here your emphasis should be on lower-body endurance. Of course, your cardio work will be taken to the extreme with long daily runs. Two full-body resistance sessions per week can definitely increase performance levels by adding some muscle to your lower body and even increasing your lung capacity. The risk of injury is also reduced as you strengthen, tone, and stretch your body.

**Q:** *I'm interested purely in burning fat and not in building muscle. Why should I strength train?*

**A:** There are two reasons. First of all, muscle tissue requires a lot of calories just to exist. This translates into a faster metabolism and more fat burning if you can put on just a little muscle. Second, the recovery from anaerobic work is an aerobic or fat burning process. So, while you're being a couch potato after your workout, you're still burning fat.

**Q:** *If I do enough sit-ups or other abdominal work, will I get a flat stomach?*

**A:** No. The reason you don't have a flat stomach has nothing to do with how many sit-ups you do. You need to do more cardio or aerobic work, burning lots of fat as well as teaching your body to be a better fat burner. Then those rock-hard abs from doing all those sit-ups will finally be visible. Another point worth mentioning is the impact a nutrition program has on body-fat percentages.

**Q:** *I'm a 35-year-old female, and I'm afraid of getting muscles. Do I need to worry?*

**A:** This is a very common concern for women attempting to get in shape. While most women may not be able to pack on the muscle mass some men can, it is a genuine concern. The answer is very simple. You are in control of the process, and if an area of your body begins to seem too overdeveloped, back off on your training for that particular muscle group. You can always do less or switch to a maintenance routine.

**Q:** *I love to run outdoors, but winter is approaching and I don't want to run in the bitter cold. What do you suggest as an alternate exercise to my outdoor jogging program?*

**A:** The answer to this question is based on three factors: (1) the monetary investment you're willing to make, (2) the space required to store a large piece of exercise equipment, and (3) personal preference. If you can afford it and have the room, I recommend a treadmill, the least gimmicky but probably the most effective piece of aerobic exercise equipment you can purchase. If you're limited on money and space, a simple jump rope can be quite effective in getting you into the target heart-rate zone. Another inexpensive alternative would be an athletic step to get you through those long, cold winter months indoors.

**Q:** *I love to run but have problems with the impact it has on my knees and lower back, causing pain and stiffness. What do you suggest?*

**A:** If it hurts, don't do it. If you've approached your training properly—that is, you've rested long enough between sessions and performed all your flexibility exercises—and you still have pain with some movements, sometimes the only thing to do is avoid those movements completely and find alternatives that work. Aerobic exercises that are low impact include cycling (indoor and on a stationary bike), low-impact aerobic classes, and even brisk walking.

**Q:** *Which gives you a more effective workout, machines or free weights?*

**A:** Your muscles cannot distinguish between sophisticated health club machines and simple dumbbells, and as long as you achieve proper form and intensity, they will respond. Machines do provide another dimension to help avoid boredom and maintain a program with a variety of movements, but they are far from vital to the process.

**Q:** *I'm too overweight to even think about exercising. How can I begin?*

**A:** If you're obese and have any health issues, please see your doctor as your first step before you start exercising. Second, just begin walking every day or every other day. Don't worry about how far or how fast you go, but try to improve slightly every couple of workouts. Most important, watch what you eat. Keep your food dense in nutrients and low in fat, but don't starve yourself. When you feel strong enough, start a beginning strength routine with light resistance.

**Q:** *Sometimes, after an exceptionally long or intense workout, I feel extremely fatigued and even experience some loss of appetite and irritability. Am I training too much?*

**A:** Everyone has a different level of energy that can be expended during a workout or series of workouts before it becomes detrimental or counterproductive to one's overall goals. This applies to your cardio program as well as your strength-training regimen. If you experience any of the listed signs or symptoms, carefully examine your exercise routine, nutrition program, and sleeping patterns to see which may be causing the problem. If the problem is excessive exercise, I suggest taking a week or two completely off. When you return to your program, ease up on the duration, frequency, and/or intensity of your routine. Remember, the actual benefits of exercise are realized during the rest periods between sessions, so give yourself plenty of rest and recuperation periods, eat right, and get adequate amounts of sleep.

Here are the classic signs of overtraining:

▶ Weight loss
▶ Appetite loss
▶ Fatigue
▶ Difficulty sleeping
▶ Lack of progress in your exercise routine
▶ Minor colds
▶ Irritability

**Q:** *As a senior citizen who's never worked out before, I'm concerned about overdoing it and injuring myself. Can I still benefit from an exercise and nutrition program?*

**A:** Everyone can benefit from working out and eating right. Youth does not have the corner on the exercise market. In fact, the muscle tissue of a 25-year-old man is identical to the muscle tissue of a 75-year-old man. Certain adjustments must be made, and often the goals of seniors may be somewhat different, but the principles still work. More rest between workouts and decreased intensity levels are usually indicated. Careful attention is paid to nutrition, flexibility movements, and sleeping habits. Cardiovascular work is done at the low end of the target heart-rate zone, and resistance work is modified to fit the individual. As we age, our bodies naturally lose bone and muscle mass. Exercise, combined with a solid nutrition program and the proper rest and recuperation, will interfere with this process.

**Q:** *Occasionally, on the day following an intense but invigorating training session, the muscle or muscles involved become sore and stiff. Is this normal, and is there any way to avoid it?*

**A:** What you're experiencing here is *delayed muscle soreness* (DMS). It's perfectly normal, especially when performing any new movements that your muscles haven't yet adapted to. Once you're at the point of feeling pain, the healing process is underway, and it should subside in 24 hours or so. To minimize any pain when performing new movements, ease up on intensity levels until your body can adapt. If the pain persists beyond a day or two, it's probably not DMS, and you should consult your doctor.

**Q:** *How can I increase the intensity of my strength-training exercises without just lifting more weight?*

**A:** With a little imagination the variations are endless. Here are a few:

▶ Increase repetitions.
▶ Decrease rest between sets.
▶ After your last set, without any rest in between, do two or three more sets with lighter weight, each set done with perfect form and to failure.
▶ Perform the set in slow motion (to a count of 4 on the exhalation and 8 on the inhalation).
▶ If you have the luxury of a trainer or a training partner, have them assist you with a few "cheating" reps.

**Q:** *When I hit the gym, I rarely have a plan but rather gravitate to whatever I feel like doing. Can I get results this way?*

**A:** If you're out of shape and have never trained before, just about anything you do will have some effect. The Firefighter's Workout delivers the maximum effectiveness for the minimum investment, because it is a sound fitness system that's also well organized and structured and doesn't waste your time, energy, and money. Planning and recording your training sessions will aid you in taking advantage of the *adaptation response*, whereby you add slight increases in intensity with each workout. Have a clear picture in your mind of where you want that workout ultimately to bring you, and you'll arrive that much sooner.

**Q:** *So much has been written about the target heart-rate zone in the last 10 years. Why is this so important?*

**A:** This is a very good question, and I'll explain what your heart rate has to do with burning fat. When you train, your body's metabolism gets revved up as it rises to meet the demands being placed upon it. One of the things it must do is supply fuel to those working muscles. During anaerobic activity (which consists of short bursts of intense movement, such as weight lifting or sprinting), primarily sugar (a small supply of which is stored in the muscle itself as glycogen) is burned. The problem with this system is that supplies run out rather quickly. However, aerobic activity (which consists of sustained motion, such as jogging or swimming) uses oxygen, sugar, and *fat* as its chief sources of fuel. Scientists have found that the body is at its most aerobic (burning oxygen, sugar, and fat) when the heart rate is at 60 to 90 percent of its maximum capacity. Above 90 percent is considered anaerobic activity, and at that level, you'll be burning mostly sugar instead of stored body fat. See Chapter 3, for more information on how to calculate your individual target heart-rate zone.

**Q:** *Should I eat before a workout?*

**A:** It's essential that you consume some calories, mostly in the form of carbohydrates, before you exercise. Whether your training session will consist mostly of strength-training or cardiovascular conditioning exercises, you'll require an adequate fuel supply to sustain the working muscles. This doesn't mean you should overeat and try to exercise while your stomach is busy digesting a heavy meal. Eat a very light carbohydrate-based snack such as dry cereal or fruit half an hour or 20 minutes before you train. After your training session, your muscles will become nutrient starved as your metabolism revs up. This is the perfect time to consume larger amounts of high-protein and -carbohydrate foods.

# PARK SLOPE

As a firefighter for 15 years, I'd performed cardiopulmonary resuscitation (CPR) many times, but as anyone who's done it knows, with limited success. In the mid-1990s, things changed considerably when the New York City fire department instituted a policy of dispatching a fire truck to all critical emergency medical calls. Each firefighter received a tremendous amount of training, and the units were equipped with defibrillators. That turned out to be a very good thing for Salvatore.

Sal was a 55-year-old guy from the old neighborhood, visiting a buddy he hadn't seen in a year or two at his local auto repair shop. The two old friends had lunch together, and as they stood on the sidewalk in front of the little shop saying their good-byes, Sal's eyes suddenly rolled back in his head, and his body collapsed like a ton of bricks.

At that moment, Sal's buddy ran back inside the shop and made a frantic call to 911. About a minute later, we were dispatched from our firehouse less than a mile away. We pulled up to a panicky scene as a dozen bystanders crowded around Sal while he lay dying in the street. I strained my eyes trying to see through the mob around Sal, and what struck me most was the color of his skin. Inhuman might be the best way to describe it. The human body changes fast when it is robbed of its blood supply with its life-giving oxygen, even momentarily. I wasn't sure how long he hadn't been breathing, but his skin was ashen gray or cyanotic, and his glassed-over eyes looked as if they were about to pop from his skull.

We jumped off the rig and scooped up our equipment. Like a scene from the television series *ER*, we all went into action. The oxygen was hooked up, the resuscitator was applied, and chest compressions were performed. We were simulating Sal's own natural breathing and heartbeat, but the man was still gray. That's when Victor, one of the firefighters working that afternoon, got the defibrillator hooked up and set to go. I heard Vic say in a loud clear voice, "Clear!"

We all dropped what we were doing, leaned away, and Victor hit the shock button. Sal's 200-plus-pound body jolted a full six inches off the ground, but the electrocardiograph (EKG) monitor on the defibrillator machine still showed no appreciable heartbeat. Again, Vic yelled "Clear!" and we all backed off. Before Sal's body had settled back onto the ground, I saw the heart monitor going up and down in a normal rhythm. I blinked my eyes and looked again, but sure enough, his heart began to beat by itself.

We continued to provide Sal with extra oxygen, but he was able to breathe on his own. By the time the medics had arrived, his skin pallor was normal, and he'd regained a small degree of consciousness. Still not quite able to speak, he looked at me with fear and confusion in his eyes. I helped him into the ambulance and said softly, "Don't worry, Salvatore, everything's gonna be okay."

I wondered if he had any idea how close he had just come to death.

# WHAT'S SO GREAT ABOUT BEING A FIREFIGHTER

They look at us with beaming cherub faces like we're larger than life. To them we're Batman and Superman all rolled into one, but in reality we're just normal guys who are ready and willing to go that extra mile when the situation calls for it.

That day we squeezed the fire truck into an oversized parking space on the bustling avenue while going about our routine duties. Inevitably a young mother, wheeling one baby and carrying the other, busy with her daily chores, was stopped dead in her tracks by her little boy, his gaze transfixed on the big red fire truck.

We always have time for children—some shy, some a little afraid, others with a thousand questions, but all barely taller than the front wheel of the fire truck. When I walked over to him and he gave me that wide-eyed look, I realized why I'd become a fireman in the first place. I knelt down to his level and asked softly, "Hey little guy, wanna ride on the fire truck?" Mom answered for him, "Of course he does, he absolutely loves firemen."

If you can go through this life and manage to get the love of children, you've accomplished something. I thought to myself, "That's why I love being one."

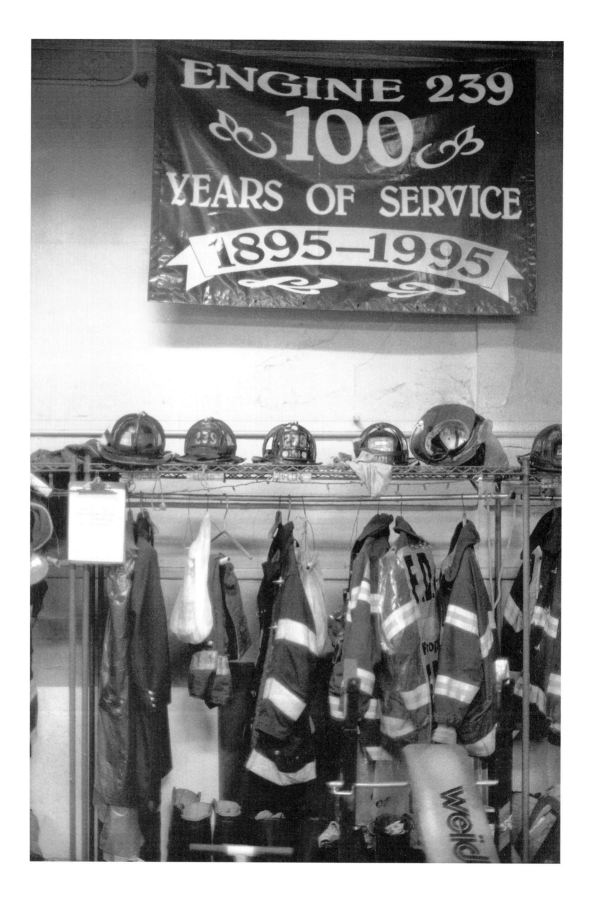

# Conclusion and Review

**F**irefighters know all too well the importance of being ready for anything. In this busy world you barely have enough time to pause and take a breath, never mind a long, draining workout. It's reassuring to know that you can get the exercise you need in a quick but intense training session that's based on sound and proven principles—a workout routine that won't drain your energy levels for hours afterward. As a matter of fact, you'll be energized and ready for anything your day has to offer after your workout is complete.

With *The Firefighter's Workout Book* it takes only a few hours a week to work your way to a fit, healthy, attractive body. Long, drawn-out hours in the gym are unnecessary and even counterproductive to your goals.

Another aspect of the program is its deemphasis of expensive equipment. A bench, a set of dumbbells, and a good pair of running shoes are all you'll need to get in the shape of your life.

All obstacles have been removed from your path and now it's time for you to do your part. A brief review of the Firefighter's Workout system follows. Good training!

## The Mental Game

▶ Decide what your goals are as they relate to *performance, appearance,* and *health.*

▶ Record your *ultimate, long-term,* and *short-term goals.*

▶ Reward yourself any time you achieve those goals.

▶ Maintain your mental focus using the simple meditation presented in Chapter 2.

▶ Learn to energize your body and your mind with proper breathing.

▶ Always pay close attention to what your body is telling you, and adjust your workout accordingly.

▶ Plan your training program and your meals in advance.

▶ Set aside time each week to meet the demands of your exercise and nutrition program.

## Cardiovascular Conditioning

▶ Pick an exercise you like that's suited to your level of fitness. Change the mode of exercise as often as you like. Besides being a great way to avoid boredom, this also helps to eliminate overuse injuries.

▶ Select proper footwear to match your activity. For example, don't wear basketball shoes to run.

▶ Warm up before and cool down after every workout.

▶ Beginners should *always* start slowly and increase their duration, frequency, and/or intensity levels gradually, avoiding overuse injuries and allowing the adaptation response to take effect.

▶ Ensure that you're in the *target heart-rate zone* by monitoring your pulse or breathing rate and using the formulas given in chapter 3. Ensure that you're in the zone for at least 15 minutes. Working at the high end of the zone (near 90 percent of your maximum heart rate [MHR]) will reduce the length of time of your training session while producing dramatic results, but progress can still be achieved at the low end.

▶ Repeat your cardio workout anywhere from two to six times per week, depending on your fitness goals. If the main thrust of your entire routine is to burn fat, repeat your aerobic workouts more often.

▶ Record your training sessions as outlined in Chapter 5.

▶ Integrate your cardiovascular training with your strength and flexibility training by using the workout routines that apply to you, as presented in Chapter 5.

▶ If you are too out of shape to do anything else, just walk. Gradually increase the length and intensity of your walks, and be sure to do pulse checks at various intervals to determine where you are in relation to the target heart-rate zone.

## Strength Training

▶ Always warm up prior to and stretch out after your resistance workout.

▶ Whether you're training with sophisticated machines or simple dumbbells, proper form and adherence to the ABCs are essential to success and injury prevention.

▶ Select a weight or resistance level that coincides with your level of fitness and allows you to hit muscle fatigue at your desired repetition range (normally either 8 to 12 or 12 to 15, depending on your goals). Gradually attempt to increase the weight from workout to workout and, if called for in the specific routine, from set to set.

▶ Heavy weight lifted for low repetitions (fewer than 8) will build more strength and mass than a lighter weight lifted for a moderate number of repetitions (8 to 15), which will build more endurance while it tightens and tones. The first warmup set should generally be 20 reps.

▶ Rest between 48 and 96 hours before retraining the same muscle or muscle group.

▶ As a general rule, rest one to two minutes between each set unless contradicted by protocol called for with a specific routine.

▶ Beginners should always start slowly, doing only as much as they can handle, gradually increasing resistance by taking advantage of the adaptation response.

▶ Vary your training program by changing exercises and routines every month or two.

▶ Record all your workouts (see Chapter 5) and use the 1-to-5 scale to rate your intensity.

▶ Ideally, your aerobic training and your strength training should be done on alternate days, but if you only have three days a week to work out, combine them. Be flexible in your scheduling.

▶ When engaging in an intense strength-training program, ensure that your body gets plenty of rest and sleep nightly.

▶ Pay attention to your body, and avoid overtraining by resting when necessary.

## Flexibility Training

▶ The flexibility segment of your workout should be done when the body is warm, preferably at the end of either the aerobic or strength segment. Stretching exercises can also be mixed in with strength movements to save time.

▶ As just stated, you cannot stretch a cold muscle—doing so will result in injury and will accomplish nothing.

▶ Static stretches should generally be held from 15 to 30 seconds. A sum total of 30 seconds is necessary to achieve any kind of permanent stretch.

▶ Generally, breathe out when going into the stretch, and inhale when coming out of it, using the breath as a way to go further into the movement.

▶ Never stretch to the point of feeling pain, just slight discomfort. If you experience pain, you're just creating more tension and risking possible injury.

▶ Unlike strength-training or intense aerobic workouts, your flexibility segment can be repeated every day. Stretching has a healing effect on the body and does not require the same recuperation period as running or lifting weights.

▶ Vary the stretching exercises from day to day to ensure hitting all areas and relieving any boredom. If you follow the routines in Chapter 5, you'll find the exercises are somewhat varied.

▶ Again, beginners should start slowly and increase the length of time stretches are held or the number of sets per workout, taking advantage of the adaptation response. Another option might be to take it a step further and take a yoga class, which makes a great adjunct to the Firefighter's Workout.

▶ The flexibility segment of your workout can make a natural cooldown period from either an intense aerobic or strength-training session.

# Nutrition

▶ Avoid unhealthy, nutrient-deficient fad diets that might rob you of lean muscle mass.

▶ Use body-fat assessment as a way to evaluate the progress of your nutrition and exercise program.

▶ Use the four-food-group system as a guide to your daily food intake.

| Group 1 | Meat | Two or three daily servings |
| Group 2 | Milk | Two or three daily servings |
| Group 3 | Grains | At least four daily servings |
| Group 4 | Vegetables | At least four daily servings |
| Nonfood group | Fats, oils, sweets | Use sparingly |

▶ Ensure that you're getting an adequate supply of protein, carbohydrates, vitamins, minerals, and fiber. If you adhere to the four-food-group system, this will happen automatically.

▶ Drink three or four quarts of water daily. Ensure that you're well hydrated before, during, and after exercise.

▶ Take a close look at what you presently eat and make every effort to improve upon that.

▶ Using one of the sample meal plan charts as a guide, record what you eat every day using a blank chart (see Appendix C).

▶ Adjust your caloric intake to fit your metabolism and activity levels.

▶ If at all possible, plan your meals in advance.

▶ This has been said thousands of times by thousands of people: Don't smoke, and drink alcohol only in moderation (a lot of hidden calories there).

▶ Get the advice of your doctor before making any major changes in your present diet.

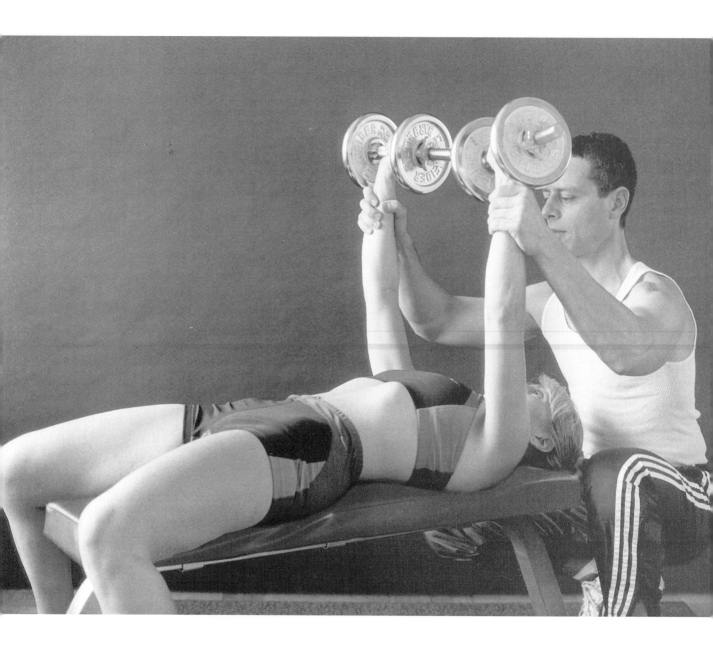

# Glossary of Common Jargon

**Y**ou hear people tossing words around the gym like a medicine ball, but you're often too embarrassed to admit your lack of knowledge. Not to worry, here are some of the most common words, slang and otherwise, that any seasoned bodybuilder could hurl at you.

**active rest**   A light workout or activity that is done at a much lower intensity level than your usual training session, thus enabling you to train but still get the recuperation period your body needs.

**adaptation response**   The body's ability to respond to any demand placed upon it by gradually growing stronger. This applies to bones, ligaments, tendons, and muscles, as well as the efficiency of the heart-lung system.

**aerobic**   "With oxygen." This is the system of energy the body uses when there is an adequate supply of oxygen available, usually when the body is working at 60 to 90 percent of full capacity, at which time the maximum amount of fat is being burned as fuel rather than carbohydrate (sugar).

**anaerobic**   "Without oxygen." This is the system of energy the body uses when there is not an adequate supply of oxygen available due to increased demand. When the body is working at above 90 percent of capacity, it burns mostly glycogen (sugar) for energy. The recovery from anaerobic exercise can be aerobic (oxygen- and fat-burning).

**body awareness**   Refers to how you carry your body through your daily activities (posture) as well as during exercise. Strengthening and stretching exercises can have a profound impact on your body awareness, and on the way you move and use your body during routine daily activities as well as during exercise.

**cheating**   Bringing other muscles or momentum (rocking back and forth) into play to complete a lift. While it may have a place for power lifters, it has limited value for body sculpting or toning, and should not be used for our purposes here. Rather, strict adherence to proper form is called for.

**circuit training**   This takes the concept of supersets or trisets even further. Here you combine multiple movements (exercises), and possibly the entire workout, one set after another, with brief or possibly no rest periods between sets (see Chapter 5, Routine 3).

**delayed muscle soreness (DMS)**    Usually experienced 24 to 48 hours after an activity in the muscle actually worked, this is a normal response to intense exercise. Once the pain is felt, the healing process has begun. This pain should be not be confused with joint, tendon, or ligament pain that could be a sign of an overuse injury, requiring some rest and recuperation.

**duration**    Length of time it takes to complete a workout or segment of a workout (see Chapter 3).

**form**    Proper form (the opposite of **cheating**) refers to performing the movement properly without using momentum or swinging or jerking motions to complete a lift, following the ABCs of strength training (see Chapter 3).

**frequency**    How often a training session is repeated (see Chapter 3).

**intensity**    In strength training, how far past muscle fatigue you're able to go, reaching total muscle failure at higher intensities. In cardio training, how far into the target heart-rate zone you're able to go. (See Chapter 3.)

**interval training**    A way of performing your cardio workout. The training session is broken down into sets of anywhere from 10 seconds to 10 minutes or more. Intensity is increased and brief active rest periods are allowed between each segment.

**modality**    The type of exercise or equipment used during the workout (see Chapter 3).

**muscle failure**    Implies that the muscle being worked can absolutely not do another repetition without abandoning proper form (**cheating**) or bringing other muscles into play.

**muscle fatigue**    As used here, *fatigue* refers to the point in the set where you begin to experience some discomfort and possible weakening of the muscle or muscle group being trained.

**negative reps**    See **positive/negative reps.**

**overtraining**    Too much of a good thing can be bad. *Overtraining* can occur on many levels, but it mostly refers to working out too much and not giving the body a chance to heal itself. All progress will be halted; other possible symptoms include loss of appetite, irritability, weight loss, injury, and insomnia.

**positive/negative reps**    Any resistance movement in strength training can be broken down into two phases; the *positive phase,* in which the weight is lifted against gravity (exhalation phase), and the *negative phase,* in which the weight is controlled as it is lowered against gravity (inhalation phase). Some researchers believe more muscle building is accomplished during the negative phase, which should be slow and controlled and should take twice as long as the positive portion of the movement.

**prone**    The opposite of **supine;** lying flat on the stomach.

**pyramid training**    Changing the amount of resistance (weight) from set to set, usually from low to high and back again (see Chapter 5).

**rep**    Repetition. Refers to the number of times a movement is repeated within each set. See **set.**

**set**    A group of repetitions performed at one time during a resistance or strength-training exercise. For example, "John did one set of 10 repetitions."

**superset**    Implies completing two separate and distinct sets one after the other without resting in between sets. A *triset* or *quadset* would imply completing three or four sets without rest.

**supine**    The position of the human body when lying flat on the back, as in a bench press.

**volume**    The number of sets or exercises performed in a given workout (see Chapter 3).

# Anatomically Correct

**T**here are five major anatomical groups within the human body, the *cardiovascular, respiratory, nervous, skeletal,* and *muscular systems,* which all work together to sustain life and move you from place to place. The heart pumps the blood that carries the oxygen and nutrients to the organs and muscles. The nervous system sends electrical signals from the brain to the muscles, making them contract. The contracting muscles, connected to the skeletal system via tendons, act upon each bone, and the end result is motion.

## The Major Muscle Groups

A basic understanding of the location and function of the major muscles and muscle groups will assist you in putting together an exercise regimen that works. For our purposes, we'll divide the body into three separate areas.

**UPPER BODY**
- Chest—pectoral muscle
- Shoulders—deltoids (front, side, and rear)
- Back—latissimus (lats) and trapezius
- Biceps (upper frontal arm)
- Triceps (upper rear arm)
- Forearm

**LOWER BODY**
- Quadriceps (upper frontal leg)
- Hamstrings (upper rear leg)
- Gluteus maximus (buttocks or glutes)
- Calves

**CORE**
- Abdominals and obliques
- Lower back (muscles surrounding the spine)

See illustrations in Figures B.1 and B.2.

**FIGURE B.1   ANATOMICAL DIAGRAM (FRONT VIEW)**

**FIGURE B.2   ANATOMICAL DIAGRAM (REAR VIEW)**

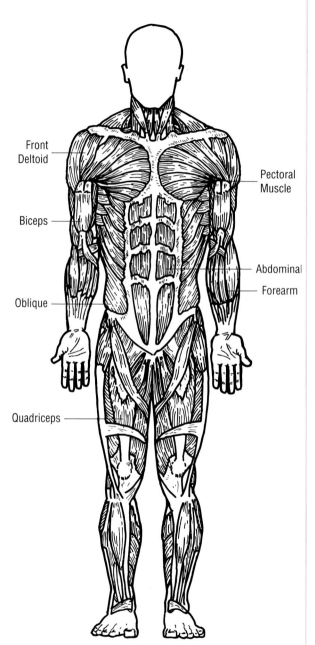

Front Deltoid

Pectoral Muscle

Biceps

Abdominal

Forearm

Oblique

Quadriceps

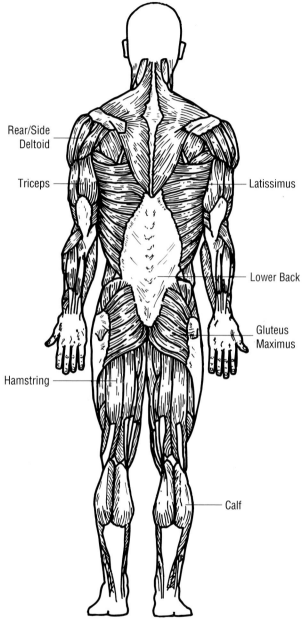

Rear/Side Deltoid

Triceps

Latissimus

Lower Back

Gluteus Maximus

Hamstring

Calf

# Blank Charts

## ULTIMATE, LONG-TERM, AND SHORT-TERM GOALS

Name                                                    Date

**ULTIMATE GOAL—PERFORMANCE**

**ULTIMATE GOAL—APPEARANCE**

**ULTIMATE GOAL—HEALTH**

**LONG-TERM GOAL—PERFORMANCE**

**LONG-TERM GOAL—APPEARANCE**

**LONG-TERM GOAL—HEALTH**

**SHORT-TERM GOAL—PERFORMANCE**

**SHORT-TERM GOAL—APPEARANCE**

**SHORT-TERM GOAL—HEALTH**

## FOUR-FOOD-GROUP MEAL PLAN

| Meal/Time | Foods | Calories | Protein (g) | Carbs (g) | Fat (g) | Food Group |
|-----------|-------|----------|-------------|-----------|---------|------------|
| BREAKFAST | | | | | | |
| | | | | | | |
| | | | | | | |
| SNACK | | | | | | |
| | | | | | | |
| | | | | | | |
| LUNCH | | | | | | |
| | | | | | | |
| | | | | | | |
| SNACK | | | | | | |
| | | | | | | |
| | | | | | | |
| DINNER | | | | | | |
| | | | | | | |
| | | | | | | |
| SNACK | | | | | | |
| | | | | | | |
| | | | | | | |
| TOTALS | | | | | | |

### Daily Comments

MEAT GROUP:

MILK GROUP:

GRAIN GROUP:

VEGETABLE GROUP:

NONFOOD GROUP (FAT/OIL/SUGAR):

## DAILY EXERCISE RECORD

**Strength Routine**

| WARMUP | MODE: | | | DURATION: | | | |
|---|---|---|---|---|---|---|---|
| **MUSCLE GROUP** | **EXERCISE** | **SET 1** | **SET 2** | **SET 3** | **SET 4** | **SET 5** | **COMMENTS** |

### Weight/Repetitions

| | | | | | | | |
|---|---|---|---|---|---|---|---|
| | | | | | | | |
| | | | | | | | |
| | | | | | | | |
| | | | | | | | |
| | | | | | | | |
| | | | | | | | |

**Flexibility Routine**

| **MUSCLE GROUP** | **EXERCISE** | **SET 1** | **SET 2** | **SET 3** | **SET 4** | **SET 5** | **COMMENTS** |
|---|---|---|---|---|---|---|---|

### Indicate a check or hold time for each set completed

| | | | | | | | |
|---|---|---|---|---|---|---|---|
| | | | | | | | |
| | | | | | | | |
| | | | | | | | |
| | | | | | | | |
| | | | | | | | |
| | | | | | | | |

| **Cardio Routine** | **Mode** | **Duration** | **Max Heart Rate** | **Comments** |
|---|---|---|---|---|
| | | | | |
| | | | | |

## FITNESS ASSESSMENT

| FITNESS TEST | DATE | DATE | DATE |
|---|---|---|---|
| Max push-up test | | | |
| 3-minute step test | | | |
| Sit-and-reach test | | | |
| **BODY COMPOSITION** | **DATE** | **DATE** | **DATE** |
| Circumference Measurements | | | |
| Upper arm | | | |
| Thigh | | | |
| Waist | | | |
| Hips | | | |
| Chest | | | |
| | | | |
| Body Weight | | | |
| | | | |
| **BODY-FAT PERCENTAGE** | | | |
| Method | | | |
| Percentage | | | |
| | | | |
| **PHYSICIAN'S SECTION** | **DATE** | **DATE** | **DATE** |
| Resting heart rate | | | |
| Max heart rate | | | |
| Blood pressure | | | |
| Cholesterol level | | | |
| Triglyceride level | | | |

# Index